The Miracle

Molecule

By

Kim Nicholson

MS., Lifestyle Medicine, B.S., Nutrition,

AAH, HWC, CHHS, AAD, DipACLM, Chef

Disclaimer

This book, "The Miracle Molecule," is intended for informational purposes only and does not serve as a substitute for professional medical advice, diagnosis, or treatment. The contents of this book, including but not limited to text, graphics, images, and other material, are for informational purposes only and not intended to be a substitute for professional medical advice or treatment. Always seek the advice of your physician or other qualified health provider with any questions you may have regarding a medical condition or health objectives.

The author and publishers are not responsible for any specific health or allergy needs that may require medical supervision and are not liable for any damages or negative consequences from any treatment, action, application, or preparation, to any person reading or following the information in this book. The information in this book is being provided without warranty of any kind, either express or implied, and is not intended to replace discussions with a healthcare provider.

All decisions regarding patient care must be made with a healthcare provider, considering the unique characteristics of the patient. The views expressed in this book are the opinions of the author and do not necessarily reflect the views of the publisher.

No part of this book should be considered or used as a substitute for professional medical advice, diagnosis, or treatment. You should not use this information to diagnose or treat a health problem or disease without consulting with a qualified healthcare provider. Please consult your healthcare provider with any questions or concerns you may have regarding your condition.

Table of Contents

Welcome to The Miracle Molecule

Hey there, amazing friends!

I'm beyond excited to bring you along on a journey that's close to my heart. We're about to explore the wonders of what I love to call "The Miracle Molecule" - yep, you guessed it, water! This isn't just any old science talk; it's a celebration of life's most essential ingredient, both in the world around us and the incredible universe within us.

Water is everywhere, from the oceans that cradle our continents to the clouds above. But the true magic? It's how water works inside us, playing a star role in every smile, every thought, and every little thing that makes us, well, us. Together, we're going to uncover not just how water shapes rivers and valleys but how it shapes you and me.

Inside every one of us, water is doing its thing - hustling oxygen to our cells, carrying away the bad stuff, and making sure the intricate dance of our bodily processes goes off without a hitch. It's like the ultimate backstage pass to the coolest show on Earth, happening right in our cells.

And here's the heart-to-heart part: water connects us to life itself. It's a reminder that we're all in this together, sharing this beautiful blue planet. By getting up close and personal with water's role in our bodies, we can't help but feel a stir to protect this precious resource that binds us all.

So, consider this book your invitation from me to you, to rekindle your awe for the liquid life force that's water. Let's celebrate its everyday miracles, from quenching our thirst to keeping the delicate balance of our bodies just right.

Thank you for being here with me. Let's get inspired, let's get connected, and let's marvel at the wonders of water, the true essence of life, that flows through us all.

With deepest appreciation and shared wonder,

Kim Nicholson

The Miracle Molecule

Water, often referred to as the elixir of life, is the cornerstone of our existence. Comprising two hydrogen atoms bonded to an oxygen atom, this seemingly simple molecule holds the key to life's complexity and diversity. Its unique molecular structure endows it with properties that are foundational to life on Earth, meriting the title of "the miracle molecule."

Water's molecular structure is a marvel of nature that underpins its life-sustaining properties. The arrangement of its atoms gives water a polar nature, allowing it to dissolve more substances than any other liquid and earn the title of "universal solvent." This capability is crucial for life on Earth, as it enables water to carry vital nutrients to cells, transport waste products away, and participate in countless biochemical reactions that keep organisms alive. Moreover, water's unique properties extend to its role in climate regulation. Its ability to absorb and retain heat stabilizes Earth's temperature, making it habitable for diverse forms of life.

Water's high specific heat capacity, latent heat of vaporization, and latent heat of fusion contribute to moderating the global climate, cushioning the planet from extreme temperature fluctuations. Water's versatility in form—as a solid (ice), liquid, and gas (water vapor)—facilitates various ecological and physiological processes. Ice's lower density compared to liquid water ensures that it floats, acting as an insulating layer that protects aquatic life during freezing temperatures. Meanwhile, water vapor plays a critical role in the water cycle, moving water from Earth's surface to the atmosphere and back, replenishing freshwater sources and maintaining the hydrological balance essential for all terrestrial and aquatic ecosystems. The cohesive and adhesive properties of water are equally significant. These allow water to move against gravity through plant stems and leaves, supporting plant life, which in turn sustains much of Earth's food web. On a cellular level, these properties are vital for transporting substances within organisms, highlighting water's indispensable role in the structural and functional integrity of cells. The essence of life that water represents is not merely in its physical presence but in the critical functions it performs across ecosystems and within organisms. Understanding water's molecular structure and unique properties sheds light on its irreplaceable role in maintaining life on Earth, emphasizing the need to cherish and conserve this vital resource.

Okay now onto you, and how water is a miracle molecule in your body!

THE FOUNTAIN OF YOUTH: A MYTH IN PLAIN SIGHT

Have you ever imagined finding the Fountain of Youth?

Since ancient times, people worldwide have been telling stories about a fountain of youth that might extend one's life. The fountain is a mythical spring that is said to bring back the youth of anyone who drinks or bathes in it. So, where can you find this fountain of youth? Look, it's not in Florida or the Caribbean Islands. Believe it or not… it's in your kitchen faucet! It's called water.

Throughout history, people have used this simple substance to stave off disease and live healthier lives. It is not just about drinking water from a specific place and becoming young again, but about how we all can fight growing old by living healthy and living ways that slow down the aging process.

Far from the magical properties of legend, it's the simple, everyday choices we make to stay hydrated that can decelerate the aging process. **Our planet, rich in countless wonders, counts water among its most precious gifts.** This fundamental element, essential for all known forms of life, shapes our world and every facet of our existence. Yet, for something so crucial, water is often overlooked. Our existence hinges on it, and our health flourishes with it. Beyond its biological importance, water sustains us in more mundane ways, cooling us down, quenching our thirst, and aiding in daily tasks.

Discovering Our Inner Miracle

For years, I struggled with lackluster skin, unrelenting fatigue, and a mind clouded by fog, until I embraced the ritual of proper hydration. It wasn't an overnight miracle, but as I consistently fueled my body with water, the changes were undeniable. My skin began to glow, shedding its previous dullness for a radiance that no cosmetic could mimic. Energy surged through me, turning what used to be sluggish mornings and afternoons into periods of productivity and vibrancy. Most astonishingly, the mental fog that had long hindered my clarity lifted, unveiling a sharpness and focus I thought were lost to me. While I can't guarantee that everyone will experience the exact transformation I did, I can confidently say that prioritizing hydration will make a profound difference in your health. Water is the cornerstone of well-being, influencing everything from our physical appearance to our mental acuity. So, while your journey with water may unfold differently, the positive impact it will have on your overall health is indisputable.

Embrace hydration as a key to unlocking a healthier, more vibrant version of yourself, this is why water is "The Miracle Molecule".

This book proposes a transformative view: water, in its essence, is the true Fountain of Youth.

By embracing a lifestyle that prioritizes hydration, we can tap into a source of health and vitality that is both ancient and profoundly simple. So, as we explore this miracle molecule and the myriad ways water benefits us, let's also consider how we might better appreciate and utilize this miraculous resource. By the end of our journey, you'll not only understand water's pivotal role in our lives but also how to harness its life-giving potential to feel younger, healthier, and more vibrant.

Let's begin by busting some myths!

Busting Water Myths with a Splash of Reality

It's the unsung hero of the wellness world, playing a starring role in everything from keeping your digestion smooth to making sure your cells are chatting it up properly. Yet, somehow, this superstar element gets sidelined more often than not. Why is that?

Hydration myths are like old wives' tales—widely circulated but not always steeped in truth. Here's the real deal on some of the most common misconceptions about drinking water:

- **Myth: "I don't need to drink water unless I'm thirsty."** Ah, thirst—the body's late-to-the-party guest. Waiting for thirst to show up before sipping on water is like waiting for your car to run out of gas before filling it up. It's better to keep the tank topped off.

- **Myth: "My coffee, soda, and food have enough water for me."** Sure, other beverages and foods can contribute to your hydration, but think of them more as side dishes. Water should be the main course. Those extras? They often bring along unwanted guests like sugar and caffeine.
- **Myth: "Too much water is a no-go, right?"** While it's true that there's such a thing as too much water, most of us aren't anywhere near that pool. It's more about finding your hydration sweet spot.
- **Myth: "Water is just for workout warriors."** Even if the most exercise you get is sprinting to catch the bus, your body still craves hydration. Water isn't just for gym buffs; it's for everyone.
- **Myth: "Bottled water is always better than tap water."** Not necessarily. Many municipal water systems provide water that's just as clean and safe as bottled water. Plus, tap water is often fortified with fluoride to help prevent tooth decay. Always check local water quality reports if you're concerned.
- **Myth: "Drinking water causes weight gain."** Water has zero calories. While you might temporarily see a higher number on the scale after chugging a lot of water, it's not fat—it's just fluid that your body will soon regulate.

- **Myth: "If I drink a lot of water, I can skip the moisturizer."** While staying hydrated can improve skin's elasticity and appearance, it doesn't replace topical moisturizers, which lock moisture into the skin.
- **Myth: "I can hydrate with sports drinks instead of water."** Sports drinks are designed to replace electrolytes lost during intense, prolonged exercise. They're not necessary for most daily hydration needs and often contain high levels of sugar and calories.

Common H2O Hurdles (and How to Leap Over Them)

Staying properly hydrated can feel like a chore, but it doesn't have to be. Overcoming common obstacles to hydration can make all the difference:

1. **"Water doesn't taste good."** Experiment with temperature! Some people prefer ice-cold water, while others enjoy it room temperature. Finding your preference can make a big difference. Wait until you see my recipes for eating your water, or my 100 ways to infuse your water, you are going to be surprised at the many ways and tastes that will keep you hydrated!
2. **"I don't want to buy bottled water."** Invest in a filter for your home tap or a filtering water bottle. Not only is this better for the environment, but it's also easier on your wallet.

3. **"I always choose sugary drinks out of habit."** Start by diluting your sugary beverages with water and gradually increase the water ratio. Your taste buds will adapt over time.
4. **"I don't like carrying a water bottle."** Find a bottle that fits your style and needs—there are countless designs, sizes, and types. Having a water bottle you love can motivate you to stay hydrated.
5. **"I can't tell when I'm hydrated."** Pay attention to your body's cues. Dark urine, dry mouth, and fatigue can all signal dehydration. Aim for light-colored urine as a sign of proper hydration.

Understanding the myths and hurdles associated with drinking water is the first step toward better hydration habits. *Now on to the next miracle of water!*

The Miracle Molecule - Unveiling the Wonders of Water

You never know the worth of water 'til the well runs dry ~T.Fuller

In life's essentials, water is unparalleled, embodying the elixir of vitality. Dubbed "The Miracle Molecule," water's simplicity belies its profound impact on health, physiology, and the sustenance of life itself. Let's take a look into the multifaceted roles of water, highlighting its critical importance across various bodily functions and establishing its rightful place at the miracle of holistic health.

The Essence of Life

Water is far more than a thirst quencher, it's the backbone of ecosystems, the pulse in our veins, and the unsung hero of our planet's biodiversity. Water's unique properties as the ultimate mixer, climate keeper, master of forms, and the great connector underscore its critical role in both the environment and our bodies.

Why Water is a Marvel in Molecule Form

1. **The Ultimate Mixer:** Picture water as the life of the party in the molecular world. It's an outstanding solvent, which means it can mix with a wide range of substances. This not only facilitates the delivery of vital nutrients and minerals throughout our bodies but also supports essential chemical reactions that keep the wheels of life turning.
2. **The Climate Keeper:** Water's ability to store heat is nothing short of super heroic. It can soak up a lot of energy without getting too hot too quickly, acting as Earth's thermostat and keeping the conditions on our planet just right for life to flourish.
3. **Master of Forms:** Water's unique party trick is its ability to exist as a solid, liquid, and gas within Earth's diverse habitats. Ice floats, ensuring our oceans and lakes don't turn into giant ice cubes, protecting the vibrant life within from being frozen solid.

4. **The Great Connector:** Thanks to water's cohesive and adhesive talents, it can stick to itself and other materials, defying gravity to climb up plant roots and stems and allowing insects to skate on its surface. This not only showcases nature's magic but is critical for life's processes from the ground up.
5. **The Essence of Us:** Water is the main ingredient in the broth of life that fills our cells. It's the stage where the drama of biochemical reactions unfolds, enabling our bodies to function, grow, and heal.
6. **The Stabilizer:** Life thrives on balance, and water is the ultimate mediator, maintaining a stable pH in organisms and ecosystems. This delicate balance is crucial for ensuring that life's biochemical symphony plays on in harmony.

The Integral Role of Water in Bodily Functions

Water plays a vital role in nearly every bodily function.

Water is not just a requirement for survival; it is a crucial player in your body's ability to function. Water has the unique ability to dissolve many different substances and transport them throughout the body. Water's surface tension allows it to grab onto and transport nutrients and minerals (like glucose) while carrying away waste material. Water is the universal solvent. Solvent, noun: A substance that can dissolve another substance. And it does this with particular ease, thanks to its chemical structure and surface tension. But wait! water's sticky character is not just valuable for the human body; Water also travels outside the human body where we need it in our atmosphere, lakes, oceans, rivers, and streams. As we breathe in air that contains water vapor, water condenses on our lips and evaporates as we exhale. It's a natural cycle at work-one of many that make life possible every day.

The total amount of water in our body is found in three central locations: within our cells (two-thirds of the water), in between cells and blood (one-third of the water), and outside our cells as interstitial fluid (less than 1% of the total).

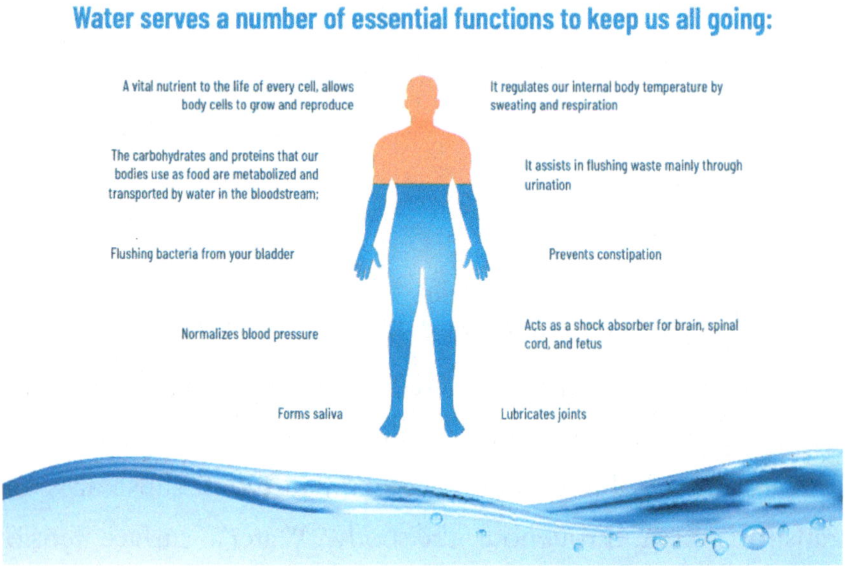

Hydration's Multidimensional Benefits

The human body, a marvel of biological engineering, is composed of approximately 60-70% water, highlighting its fundamental role in our overall health. This water is not stationary; it is in perpetual motion, circulating through our cells, organs, and tissues, facilitating a myriad of physiological functions essential for life. It transports nutrients and oxygen to cells, supports digestion, maintains blood pressure, lubricates joints, and aids in cellular metabolism, among other critical roles.

The Miracle Molecule in Action

Water's role in the body transcends mere hydration. It is integral in dissolving and transporting various substances, a property indispensable for nearly every bodily function. In the bloodstream, water transports oxygen, glucose, and lipids to cells, while also carrying away waste products to be excreted. This universal solvent capability ensures that nutrients and minerals are readily available for cellular processes and that toxins are efficiently removed, safeguarding health.

Beyond its vital role in hydration, water contributes significantly to joint health by acting as a lubricant, thus preventing the wear and tear associated with movement. It also plays a crucial role in maintaining skin health by ensuring proper hydration, which can lead to clearer, more resilient skin. In the digestive system, water aids in breaking down food, facilitating the absorption of nutrients, and promoting regular bowel movements. Furthermore, water acts as a shock absorber for the brain and spinal cord and for a developing fetus in the womb, protecting these vital structures from harm caused by sudden movements or impacts.

Maintaining the Miracle

Maintaining an optimal balance of water in the body is crucial for health and disease prevention. This balance is a dynamic process, influenced by factors such as age, activity level, climate, and individual health conditions. Recognizing the importance of hydration, experts recommend paying attention to the body's hydration cues, such as thirst and the color of urine, which should be pale yellow, indicating proper hydration.

Individual hydration needs can vary significantly, highlighting the importance of tailoring water intake to one's specific requirements. Besides drinking water, hydration can also be achieved through the consumption of food with high water content, such as fruits and vegetables. These natural sources of water can contribute significantly to daily hydration needs, offering the added benefits of nutrients and fiber.

The Integral Role of Water in Bodily Functions

Water is the cornerstone of life, it is pivotal in the transportation of nutrients and oxygen, ensuring that every cell receives the essential elements needed for energy production and overall health. This transportation system also facilitates the removal of carbon dioxide and metabolic wastes from cells, preventing toxic accumulation.

Digestion is another critical process heavily reliant on water. From the moment food enters the mouth, water works to facilitate its breakdown and absorption. Saliva, which is largely water, begins the digestive process, while water in the digestive tract aids in the dissolution of nutrients, allowing for their absorption into the bloodstream. Moreover, water is crucial in maintaining the body's temperature. Through perspiration, water evaporates from the skin's surface, dissipating heat and regulating body temperature in response to environmental and physiological factors.

Water's impact on blood health is profound. It constitutes a significant portion of blood volume, which is crucial for maintaining blood pressure within a healthy range. Proper hydration ensures that blood retains its fluidity, essential for efficient circulation and oxygen delivery. Conversely, dehydration can lead to increased blood viscosity, imposing additional strain on the cardiovascular system and potentially leading to hypertension.

Water and Electrolytes: A Harmonious Relationship

The symbiotic relationship between water and electrolytes is integral to the body's homeostasis. Electrolytes, including sodium, potassium, calcium, and magnesium, rely on water to dissolve and transport them to where they are needed, maintaining the electrical and chemical gradients crucial for life. Electrolytes play a pivotal role in fluid balance, ensuring that water is distributed appropriately across cell membranes, maintaining cell integrity and function. They are also vital for muscle contractions, including the heart muscle, enabling movement and supporting cardiovascular health. Moreover, electrolytes contribute to the regulation of the body's pH balance, ensuring that enzymatic and metabolic processes occur under optimal conditions.

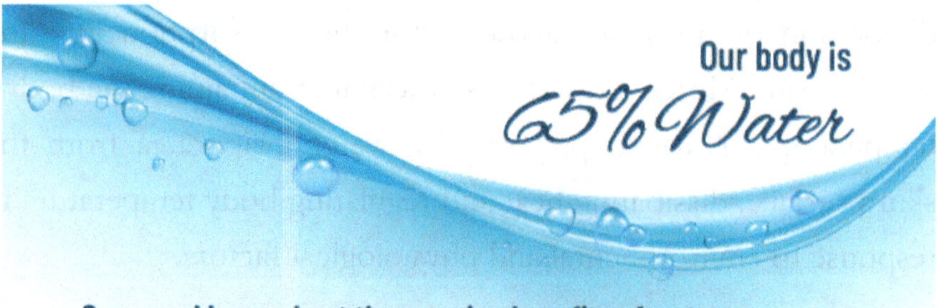

Come and learn about the amazing benefits of water.

Water is an integral part of your overall health, and a key contributor to your body's functions.
The reason different organs in the human body have different percentages of water is their different functions. Because two-thirds of total body water is contained inside cells, organs that are large and highly cellular contain a higher percentage of total body water.
The amount of water in the body changes slightly with age, sex, and hydration levels.

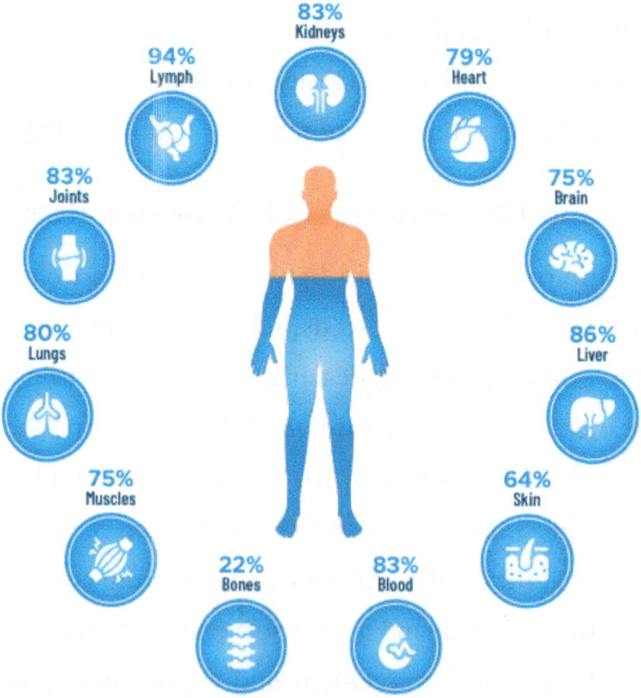

Water's Pivotal Role in Organ Functions

Water is indispensable to organ functions, particularly the kidneys, liver, and lymphatic system. The kidneys utilize water to filter blood, removing waste products and excess substances, which are then excreted as urine. Adequate hydration is essential for this filtration process, preventing kidney stones and supporting the body's detoxification processes.

The liver, another vital organ, relies on water to metabolize fats, carbohydrates, and proteins, detoxify blood, and produce bile. Water aids in these processes by facilitating the transport of nutrients and the removal of toxins from the body.

Furthermore, the lymphatic system, which is part of the body's immune defense, depends on water for the flow of lymph—a fluid that carries immune cells and waste products. Proper hydration supports lymph flow, ensuring efficient waste removal and immune function.

In the digestive system, water is crucial for breaking down food, absorbing nutrients, and eliminating waste. It supports metabolism by participating in biochemical reactions that generate energy. Thus, maintaining optimal hydration is not only vital for the health and function of specific organs but is also essential for digestion, metabolism, and waste removal processes that underpin overall health and well-being.

Water and Body Systems: Muscles, Joints, and Bones

Hydration exerts a profound influence on the musculoskeletal system, impacting muscle function, joint health, and bone integrity. Water constitutes about 75% of muscle tissue, highlighting its critical role in maintaining muscle health and function. Adequate hydration is essential for optimal muscle performance, as water facilitates the transport of nutrients to muscle cells, supports energy production, and aids in the removal of metabolic waste products. When dehydrated, muscles may experience cramps, fatigue, and reduced strength and endurance, impacting physical performance adversely.

Joints, the connectors between bones that allow for smooth movement, rely on hydration for their lubrication. Synovial fluid, a viscous liquid that reduces friction between joint surfaces, is primarily made of water. Proper hydration ensures that this fluid maintains its lubricating properties, thereby preventing joint stiffness and reducing the risk of wear and tear. Additionally, hydrated cartilage, which pads the joints, is more resilient and better able to absorb shock, minimizing the risk of joint injuries.

Bones, though seemingly rigid structures, also benefit from hydration. Water contributes to the maintenance of bone density and strength by supporting the transportation of essential minerals, such as calcium, into bone tissue. Moreover, adequate hydration can aid in the prevention of conditions like osteoporosis by ensuring a balance of nutrients that are vital for bone health.

The impact of hydration extends to physical performance and recovery. During physical activity, muscles generate heat, which the body dissipates through sweating—a process that relies heavily on water. Adequate hydration before, during, and after exercise ensures effective thermoregulation, preventing overheating and enabling sustained performance. Furthermore, water supports the body's recovery process post-exercise by facilitating the removal of toxins and the repair of muscle tissues.

Hydration plays a pivotal role in the health and function of muscles, joints, and bones, significantly impacting physical performance and recovery. Ensuring adequate water intake is crucial for the lubrication of joints, the maintenance of muscle and bone health, and the overall optimization of the musculoskeletal system's functionality.

Water as a Shield: Protecting the Immune System and More

Hydration serves as a foundational defense mechanism, bolstering the immune system and mitigating the risk of chronic diseases. By facilitating the removal of toxins and waste products through the kidneys, liver, and sweat, adequate water intake ensures that harmful substances are efficiently expelled from the body. This detoxification process is crucial for preventing the accumulation of toxins that can weaken the immune system and increase vulnerability to infections and diseases.

Water's role in immune function extends beyond detoxification. It is essential for the production of lymph, a fluid that circulates through the lymphatic system, transporting immune cells throughout the body. These cells are tasked with identifying and combating pathogens, such as bacteria and viruses. Hydration ensures that lymph maintains an optimal consistency, promoting the effective circulation of these vital immune cells and enhancing the body's ability to fend off infections.

Moreover, hydration influences the mucosal lining of the respiratory and digestive tracts, which act as the first line of defense against pathogens. Adequate hydration ensures these barriers are moist and intact, preventing the entry of harmful substances into the body. Furthermore, water aids in the production of saliva and tears, which contain antimicrobial properties that help reduce the risk of infections.

The protective benefits of hydration extend to the prevention of chronic diseases. Adequate water intake has been associated with a reduced risk of conditions such as urinary tract infections, kidney stones, hypertension, and certain types of cancer. By supporting the body's natural regulatory and repair mechanisms, water plays a vital role in maintaining cardiovascular health, promoting healthy kidney function, and potentially reducing the risk of cancer by diluting and flushing out carcinogens.

Water acts as a shield, not only enhancing immune function and facilitating the removal of toxins but also reducing the risk of chronic diseases. Ensuring adequate hydration is a simple yet effective strategy for enhancing overall health, underscoring the importance of water as a cornerstone of a healthy lifestyle. By maintaining hydration, individuals can support their body's defenses, promoting resilience against infections, diseases, and contributing to long-term well-being.

Key Takeaways

1. **Hydration is Fundamental to Health**: Water's role in maintaining health and preventing disease cannot be overstated. It is essential for the proper functioning of every cell, tissue, and organ in the body.
2. **Supports Detoxification and Immune Function**: Adequate hydration facilitates the removal of toxins and supports a robust immune system, reducing the risk of infections and some chronic diseases.
3. **Regulates Vital Bodily Functions**: From regulating body temperature and blood pressure to supporting digestion and nutrient transport, water is at the heart of physiological homeostasis.
4. **Enhances Physical Performance and Recovery**: Hydration is crucial for maintaining muscle function, joint lubrication, and overall physical performance. It aids in recovery and reduces the risk of injury during physical activity.
5. **Reduces the Risk of Chronic Diseases**: Regular water intake is associated with a lower risk of developing conditions such as urinary tract infections, kidney stones, hypertension, and certain cancers.

The Essential Role of Hydration in Skincare

The human skin, the largest organ, consists of cells that need water for optimal functioning. Water assists in expelling toxins and bacteria from your body, thus lowering the chances of skin issues. Therefore, if your body lacks adequate water, it affects your general health and skin, leading to problems such as breakouts, wrinkles, dullness, and puffiness.

Understanding Skin's Structure and Hydration's Role

The skin, serves as the ultimate barrier and protector against external elements. Its health, resilience, and appearance are directly influenced by hydration. The skin is anatomically structured into three primary layers, each playing a crucial role in skin health and relying on water to function optimally.

Epidermis: The Shield The outermost layer, the epidermis, acts as the skin's first line of defense against environmental aggressors such as pollutants, UV radiation, and pathogens. It comprises several sub-layers, with keratinocytes being the most prevalent cells, forming a waterproof barrier that retains moisture and keeps harmful substances at bay. Hydration plays a vital role in maintaining this barrier's integrity. Adequate water intake ensures the epidermis remains pliable and resilient, facilitating its regenerative processes and aiding in the healthy turnover of skin cells. This not only prevents dryness and flakiness but also contributes to a smooth, radiant complexion.

Dermis: The Support System Beneath the epidermis lies the dermis, a thicker layer housing the bulk of the skin's water content. This layer is rich in collagen and elastin fibers, which give the skin its elasticity and strength. The dermis also contains blood vessels, nerves, hair follicles, and sweat and oil glands, which play integral roles in skin health. Hydration is crucial here for several reasons. Firstly, water helps to transport nutrients and oxygen to the dermis, nourishing the skin cells. Secondly, a well-hydrated dermis supports the skin's elasticity, reducing the appearance of wrinkles and fine lines. Finally, hydration aids in the efficient functioning of sweat and oil glands, helping to regulate skin temperature and moisture levels.

Hypodermis: The Insulator The deepest layer, the hypodermis or subcutaneous layer, acts as a cushion, providing thermal insulation and absorbing shocks from external impacts. Composed primarily of fat cells, it also serves as an energy reserve.

Water in the hypodermis helps maintain the layer's volume and suppleness, contributing to the skin's overall firmness and contour.

The Impact of Hydration on Skin Health and Appearance Hydration's influence on skin health extends beyond mere surface level. Proper hydration:

- **Enhances Skin Elasticity**: Sufficient water intake ensures the skin remains elastic and bouncy, reducing the likelihood of developing wrinkles and sagging.
- **Improves Complexion**: Hydrated skin appears more vibrant and luminous, whereas dehydration can lead to a dull, tired-looking complexion.
- **Promotes Skin Regeneration**: Water facilitates the removal of toxins and supports cellular health, aiding in the skin's natural healing and regeneration processes.
- **Maintains Skin Balance**: Adequate hydration helps balance oil production and moisture levels, preventing issues like dryness, oiliness, or acne.

Scientific Evidence on Hydration's Impact on Skin Health

A myriad of studies and clinical research has elucidated the pivotal role of hydration in skin health. For instance, research published in the *International Journal of Cosmetic Science* has demonstrated that increasing water intake can significantly enhance the skin's hydration levels, leading to improved skin elasticity and a reduction in the visibility of fine lines and wrinkles. Furthermore, a study featured in "Clinical, Cosmetic and

Investigational Dermatology" revealed that participants who increased their water consumption noticed a marked improvement in skin hydration, which contributed to a more vibrant and youthful complexion.

These findings are supported by dermatological research indicating that hydrated skin is less prone to developing dryness, scaling, and flakiness, conditions that can exacerbate the appearance of aging. Additionally, proper hydration has been shown to bolster the skin's barrier function, enhancing its ability to retain moisture and protect against environmental stressors.

Physiological Mechanisms of Hydration in Skin Health

At the heart of hydration's benefits for skin health are several key physiological processes:

1. **Nutrient Transport and Waste Removal**: Water is crucial for the circulatory system's effective transport of nutrients to the skin and the removal of toxins and waste products. Well-hydrated skin cells can better utilize the nutrients delivered to them, promoting cell growth and renewal, while efficient waste removal helps prevent cellular damage and aging.
2. **Regulation of Body Temperature**: Water plays a vital role in the body's thermoregulation processes. Through perspiration, the body releases excess heat, with evaporating sweat helping to cool the skin and maintain an optimal internal temperature. This thermoregulatory

process is critical for preventing overheating and protecting skin cells from heat-induced stress and damage. Moreover, adequate hydration ensures that the sweat produced is less concentrated with salts and minerals, which can irritate the skin or clog pores if left to accumulate.

3. **Skin Elasticity and Volume**: Hydration directly influences the skin's elasticity and volume. Water content within the skin cells helps to plump them up, making the skin appear more firm and elastic. This volumizing effect not only reduces the appearance of wrinkles but also contributes to a smoother, more supple skin texture.
4. **Barrier Function and Hydration**: The skin's barrier function, which protects against external irritants and pathogens, relies on sufficient hydration to remain intact and effective. A well-hydrated skin barrier is better equipped to lock in moisture, maintain pH balance, and ward off infections, ensuring the skin remains healthy and resilient.

Hydration and the Body's Detoxification Process

Water is instrumental in facilitating the body's natural detoxification systems, including the liver, kidneys, and the skin itself. By promoting efficient blood circulation, water ensures the transport of nutrients to skin cells while facilitating the removal of waste products and toxins. When the body is adequately hydrated, the kidneys efficiently filter out waste products from the blood for elimination. Similarly, hydration supports the liver's ability to detoxify blood, which in turn reduces the burden of toxin removal on the skin.

Moreover, water is essential for the production of sweat, a primary means through which the body excretes toxins. Sweating not only helps to cool the body but also enables the removal of toxins through the pores. Proper hydration ensures that the sweat produced is less concentrated, minimizing the risk of clogging pores and potentially leading to skin issues like acne and breakouts.

Impact of Environmental Toxins on Skin Health

Environmental toxins, including pollutants, chemicals, and UV radiation, can have detrimental effects on skin health. These toxins can penetrate the skin barrier, leading to oxidative stress, inflammation, and the degradation of collagen and elastin. The result is premature aging, characterized by wrinkles, fine lines, and a loss of skin elasticity. Additionally, exposure to environmental toxins can exacerbate skin conditions such as eczema, psoriasis, and acne.

Strategies to Minimize the Effects of Environmental Toxins

To combat the impact of environmental toxins on the skin, a multifaceted approach is essential. Key strategies include:

1. **Maintain Adequate Hydration**: Drinking sufficient water helps to flush toxins from the body, supports skin

hydration, and aids in maintaining a healthy skin barrier capable of resisting the penetration of pollutants.

2. **Antioxidant-Rich Diet**: Consuming foods high in antioxidants can counteract the effects of oxidative stress caused by environmental toxins. Vitamins C and E, for example, help protect the skin cells from damage and support the skin's natural repair mechanisms.
3. **Regular Cleansing**: A consistent skincare routine that includes cleansing helps remove pollutants and toxins that accumulate on the skin's surface. Gentle exfoliation can also aid in unclogging pores and removing dead skin cells, enhancing the skin's detoxification process.
4. **Protective Measures**: Using skincare products that contain ingredients like antioxidants can offer additional protection against environmental stressors. Sunscreen is essential for protecting the skin from UV radiation, a significant source of free radicals.
5. **Limit Exposure**: Whenever possible, minimize exposure to known environmental pollutants. This may involve using air purifiers indoors and choosing skin care and household products that are free from harmful chemicals.

Function and Significance of the Skin Barrier

The primary function of the skin barrier is to protect the body from environmental aggressors such as pathogens, chemicals, pollutants, and physical harm. It also prevents excessive water loss, maintaining the body's hydration balance essential for all physiological processes. This protective layer is composed of dead skin cells (corneocytes) bound together by lipids, which together form a tight, protective matrix.

This barrier is significant for several reasons:

- **Defense Against Pathogens**: It serves as the first line of defense against bacterial, viral, and fungal infections.
- **Protection from Environmental Damage**: It shields the skin from the harmful effects of UV radiation, pollution, and other environmental stressors that can lead to premature aging and skin diseases.
- **Prevention of Transepidermal Water Loss (TEWL)**: It helps maintain skin hydration by preventing the evaporation of water from the skin's surface, crucial for skin health and elasticity.

Impact of Hydration on the Skin Barrier

Hydration plays a pivotal role in maintaining the integrity and functionality of the skin barrier. Proper hydration ensures that the barrier remains flexible, resilient, and effective in its protective roles. Here's how hydration influences the skin barrier:

- **Strengthens Barrier Function**: Adequate hydration helps to maintain the lipid matrix's structure, which seals the gaps between skin cells and prevents the penetration of harmful substances and excessive moisture loss.

- **Enhances Resilience**: Well-hydrated skin is more pliable and less likely to crack or break. This prevents the formation of micro-tears through which pathogens and irritants can enter, reducing the risk of infections and irritations.
- **Supports Skin Cell Renewal**: Hydration facilitates the natural shedding (desquamation) process of the stratum corneum and the subsequent renewal of the skin barrier. This renewal process is essential for the barrier's continuous repair and maintenance.
- **Regulates pH Balance**: The skin barrier's optimal functioning is maintained at a slightly acidic pH, which is supported by proper hydration. This acidity helps inhibit the growth of harmful bacteria and maintains the skin's microbiome balance.

Strategies to Support the Skin Barrier through Hydration

Maintaining the skin barrier's health involves more than just drinking water. It requires a holistic approach that includes:

- **Using Gentle Skincare Products**: Opt for skincare products designed to support the skin barrier, containing ingredients like ceramides, fatty acids, and cholesterol that mimic the skin's natural lipids.
- **Avoiding Harsh Cleansers**: Steer clear of skincare products with harsh surfactants that can strip the skin of its natural oils and weaken the skin barrier.

- **Applying Moisturizers**: Moisturizers help lock in hydration and reinforce the skin's barrier function by providing the necessary lipids to repair and strengthen it.
- **Protecting the Skin**: Use sunscreen daily to protect the skin from UV damage, and consider wearing protective clothing or seeking shade during peak sun hours.

Water's Influence on Collagen Production

Collagen, the most abundant protein in the human body, plays a crucial role in maintaining skin structure, elasticity, and youthfulness. Its production is a complex process influenced by various factors, including hydration levels in the body. Understanding water's role in collagen synthesis highlights its significance in preserving skin's elasticity and mitigating signs of aging.

The Role of Water in Collagen Synthesis

Water is indispensable for the biochemical reactions that occur in the body, including those involved in collagen production. Collagen synthesis requires a well-hydrated environment for several reasons:

- **Facilitation of Biochemical Reactions**: Collagen production involves a sequence of enzymatic reactions that occur more efficiently in a hydrated state. Water acts as a solvent, allowing reactants to meet, interact, and form collagen fibers.

- **Transportation of Nutrients**: Adequate hydration ensures the efficient transport of essential nutrients and amino acids, such as proline and lysine, to fibroblast cells responsible for collagen synthesis. These nutrients are vital precursors in the collagen production process.
- **Detoxification and Cellular Health**: Water aids in flushing toxins from the body, thereby reducing oxidative stress on cells, including fibroblasts. A clean, toxin-free environment supports the optimal functioning of these cells, enhancing their ability to produce collagen.

Vitamin C's Efficacy and Hydration

Vitamin C is a critical co-factor in collagen synthesis, aiding in the hydroxylation of proline and lysine, two amino acids essential for forming stable collagen fibers. Research has shown that vitamin C's effectiveness in promoting collagen production is significantly enhanced by adequate hydration. For instance, studies highlighted by Pullar, J.M., Carr, A.C., & Vissers, M. (2017) in the context of skin health have demonstrated that hydration levels can influence how effectively vitamin C performs its role in the collagen synthesis pathway.

Hydrated skin cells are better equipped to utilize vitamin C, ensuring its availability for collagen production. Furthermore, water helps to dissolve vitamin C, facilitating its absorption and transport to the skin cells where it is needed most. This synergy between hydration and vitamin C intake underscores the importance of consuming sufficient water alongside a diet rich in this vital nutrient to support collagen production.

Implications for Skin Health

The interplay between hydration, vitamin C, and collagen production has profound implications for skin health. Adequate hydration, coupled with sufficient vitamin C intake, can lead to more efficient collagen production, which in turn contributes to:

- **Increased Skin Elasticity**: Enhanced collagen production supports the skin's structure, improving its elasticity and reducing sagging.
- **Reduced Signs of Aging**: By maintaining the skin's collagen levels, hydration and vitamin C can diminish the appearance of wrinkles and fine lines, leading to a more youthful complexion.
- **Improved Skin Repair and Renewal**: Collagen is vital for the repair of damaged skin tissues. Optimal collagen production facilitated by proper hydration and vitamin C intake can accelerate skin healing and renewal.

Consequences of Dehydration on Skin Health

Dehydration, a condition resulting from inadequate intake or retention of water, can have far-reaching consequences on skin health, affecting its appearance, texture, and overall function. The skin, reliant on sufficient hydration to maintain its protective and regenerative capabilities, suffers noticeably when water levels in the body drop.

Immediate Impacts of Dehydration on Skin

The skin's immediate response to dehydration includes a range of undesirable changes that can significantly affect its appearance and feel:

- **Dullness and Lack of Radiance**: One of the first signs of dehydration is a noticeable loss of skin's natural luminosity, resulting in a dull, tired appearance. Hydrated skin reflects light more effectively, contributing to a vibrant, healthy glow that diminishes with dehydration.
- **Increased Sensitivity**: Dehydration compromises the skin's barrier function, making it more susceptible to irritants, allergens, and environmental stressors. This can lead to heightened sensitivity, redness, and irritation, as the skin lacks the necessary moisture to maintain its protective lipid barrier.
- **Susceptibility to Skin Disorders**: The weakened barrier function associated with dehydration also opens the door to various skin disorders. Conditions such as eczema, psoriasis, and acne may flare up more frequently or become more severe, as the skin struggles to defend against pathogens and regulate inflammation without adequate hydration.

Visible Signs of Dehydrated Skin

Dehydrated skin manifests several visible signs that can be easily observed:

- **Fine Lines and Wrinkles**: Dehydration diminishes the skin's plumpness, making fine lines and wrinkles more pronounced. The skin's surface becomes creased more easily, reflecting the lack of volume that adequately hydrated skin cells would otherwise provide.
- **Tightness and Flakiness**: Without sufficient moisture, the skin can feel uncomfortably tight and may exhibit flakiness or peeling, indicative of the loss of surface cells that cannot be effectively shed or replaced in a dehydrated state.
- **Rough Texture**: The smooth, supple texture characteristic of well-hydrated skin gives way to a rough, uneven feel as dehydration takes hold. This texture change is a direct consequence of the skin's inability to maintain proper moisture levels.

Practical Hydration Tips for Skin Care

Maintaining optimal skin health transcends the use of topical treatments and skincare products; it fundamentally begins with internal hydration. Adequate water intake is crucial for nourishing the skin from the inside out, supporting its natural functions, and preserving its vitality and youthfulness. Here are practical guidelines to ensure you're meeting your hydration needs for radiant skin.

Ensuring Adequate Daily Water Intake

- **Monitor Your Intake**: Aim for at least 8-10 glasses of water daily, adjusting based on your activity level, climate, and individual health needs. Remember, if you're active or live in a hot environment, your body will require additional fluids to compensate for the loss through sweat.
- **Set Reminders**: In today's busy world, it's easy to forget to drink water. Set reminders on your phone or use a water intake app to prompt you to hydrate regularly throughout the day.
- **Carry a Water Bottle**: Having a water bottle at hand encourages frequent sips, ensuring you stay hydrated. Opt for a reusable bottle to keep track of how much you're drinking and contribute to environmental conservation.
- **Flavor Your Water**: If plain water doesn't appeal to you, enhance its flavor with natural additions like slices of lemon, cucumber, or berries. Not only does this make hydration more enjoyable, but it also adds a nutritional boost to your water.

Incorporating High-Water-Content Foods

- **Eat Your Water**: Consuming fruits and vegetables with high water content is an excellent way to boost hydration. Watermelon, cucumber, strawberries, oranges, and leafy greens are not only hydrating but also packed with vitamins and antioxidants that benefit the skin.

- **Smoothies and Juices**: Incorporating smoothies and fresh juices into your diet can provide hydration along with a concentration of skin-loving nutrients. Just be mindful of the sugar content in fruit juices and opt for homemade versions when possible.

Utilizing Hydrating Skincare Products

- **Select Hydrating Ingredients**: Look for skincare products formulated with hydrating ingredients such as hyaluronic acid, glycerin, and aloe vera. These ingredients help attract and retain moisture in the skin, enhancing its hydration levels.
- **Layer Your Products**: Apply products from thinnest to thickest consistency to maximize absorption. For instance, start with a hydrating toner or essence, follow up with a serum rich in hyaluronic acid, and seal everything in with a moisturizer.
- **Don't Skip the Night Cream**: Nighttime is when the skin undergoes repair and regeneration. Using a hydrating night cream can provide your skin with the moisture it needs to facilitate these processes, leading to plumper, smoother skin by morning.
- **Consider a Humidifier**: If you live in a dry climate or use heating or air conditioning that dries out the air, a humidifier can add much-needed moisture to your

environment, preventing your skin from becoming dehydrated.

The Dehydrating Effects of Alcohol on Skin Health

Alcohol consumption has a diuretic effect, leading to increased urination and, subsequently, dehydration if fluid intake isn't adequately increased to compensate. This dehydration extends to the skin, which can become dry, lackluster, and less elastic due to the loss of moisture. Over time, the repeated dehydrating effect of alcohol can contribute to the accelerated appearance of aging, making fine lines and wrinkles more pronounced.

How Sugar-Laden Drinks Exacerbate Skin Aging

Sugar-laden drinks not only contribute to overall health issues but also have a specific impact on skin aging. The process of glycation, where sugar molecules attach to and damage proteins like collagen and elastin, is exacerbated by high sugar intake. These proteins are vital for keeping the skin firm and elastic. Glycation leads to the formation of advanced glycation end-products (AGEs), which can accelerate skin aging, promoting stiffness and reducing elasticity. Thus, reducing the intake of sugary beverages is crucial for maintaining skin health and preventing premature aging.

Incorporating Exfoliation and Humidification

Exfoliation is an integral part of any skincare routine, promoting the removal of dead skin cells and facilitating healthy skin turnover. However, it's crucial to approach exfoliation with balance to avoid damaging the skin's moisture barrier. Gentle exfoliation can enhance the skin's ability to retain hydration by removing the outermost layer of dead skin cells that can prevent moisturizers from penetrating deeply. Chemical exfoliants like alpha hydroxy acids (AHAs) or physical exfoliants with fine particles can be effective, provided they're used in moderation—typically, no more than once or twice a week.

Humidifiers for Skin Moisture Levels

Humidifiers are an excellent tool to improve skin moisture, particularly in environments where air is dry—due to climate, central heating, or air conditioning. By adding moisture to the air, humidifiers help prevent the skin from becoming dehydrated, which can lead to tightness, flakiness, and accentuated wrinkles. Sleeping with a humidifier can particularly benefit the skin, as it can prevent the dry air from drawing moisture away from the skin during the night.

Differentiating Humectants and Emollients

Humectants and emollients are two types of ingredients commonly found in skincare products, each playing a unique role in skin hydration.

- **Humectants** such as glycerin, hyaluronic acid, and propylene glycol work by attracting water from the atmosphere and the deeper layers of the skin to the outer layer of the skin. They are particularly beneficial in humid environments where they can draw in external moisture to hydrate the skin.

- **Emollients** like shea butter, squalane, and plant oils, on the other hand, work by filling in gaps between skin cells with lipids, creating a smooth, soft surface. They help to lock in moisture and reinforce the skin's barrier, preventing water loss.

Common Skincare Humectants and Emollients

Common Humectants:

- Glycerin: Helps to draw in and bind water to the skin, keeping it hydrated and supple.
- Hyaluronic Acid: Known for holding up to 1000 times its weight in water, it deeply hydrates the skin layers.
- Aloe Vera: Besides its humectant properties, it soothes and nourishes the skin.

Common Emollients:

- Jojoba Oil: Mirrors the skin's natural oils and deeply moisturizes without clogging pores.
- Ceramides: Lipid molecules that are naturally present in the skin, essential for maintaining the barrier and retaining moisture.
- Dimethicone: A silicone-based polymer that forms a protective coating on the skin, preventing moisture loss.

Foundational Role of Water in Brain Health

Water is the cornerstone of brain health, playing a multifaceted and vital role in its functioning:

- **Structural Integrity**: Our brains are about 75% water, and this high water content is essential for maintaining the structural integrity of brain cells. Proper hydration ensures that neurons retain their size and shape, which is crucial for forming healthy neural connections.
- **Nutrient Delivery**: Water serves as a vital medium for delivering essential nutrients to the brain. These nutrients are necessary for brain metabolism, and without an adequate supply of water, the transportation and absorption of these nutrients can be compromised.

- **Waste Elimination**: The brain generates metabolic waste as it functions, and water is key in flushing these toxins out. The brain's glymphatic system, active during sleep, uses water in the form of cerebrospinal fluid to clear away waste, including harmful proteins associated with Alzheimer's.
- **Neurotransmitter and Energy Production**: Water facilitates the production of neurotransmitters and energy within brain cells. Dehydration can lead to imbalances in neurotransmitter production, affecting mood and cognitive functions.
- **Thermal Regulation**: Water helps maintain brain temperature through its high heat capacity and by enabling sweat and evaporation, protecting the brain from overheating, which can adversely affect its function.

In summary, water is a fundamental molecule that supports the brain's health and its cognitive and emotional functions. Regular and adequate hydration is thus essential for a well-functioning brain, influencing everything from thought processes to emotional well-being.

Cognitive Performance and Hydration

Hydration exerts a significant influence on the cognitive performance of the brain, affecting various mental processes:

- **Mental Clarity and Function**: Sufficient hydration is pivotal for the brain's overall mental clarity and function. A hydrated brain can perform cognitive tasks with greater efficiency and accuracy, which is essential for learning, memory, and complex thought processes.

- **Impact of Mild Dehydration**: Even mild dehydration can lead to a decline in cognitive abilities. Research has shown that a loss of just 1-2% of body weight due to fluid loss can impair attention, short-term memory, and other cognitive functions. This highlights the importance of regular water intake to maintain cognitive performance.
- **Mood and Concentration**: Hydration levels can also impact mood and concentration. Dehydration can trigger the release of cortisol, a stress hormone, which can lead to feelings of anxiety and negatively affect concentration levels. Adequate water intake helps to balance mood and maintain focus.
- **Anxiety and Fatigue**: Dehydration can contribute to increased feelings of anxiety and fatigue. As the brain struggles to perform optimally without enough water, individuals may experience heightened stress and a reduction in energy levels, further affecting their ability to think and process information.
- **Sleep Quality**: Good hydration contributes to better sleep quality, which is inextricably linked to cognitive function. Disruptions in sleep due to dehydration can affect brain health and lead to cognitive decline over time.

Maintaining proper hydration is, therefore, not just a matter of physical health, but is intimately connected to cognitive health and the effective functioning of the brain. Regular water intake is essential to support cognitive processes that the brain undertakes every second of our lives.

Neurotransmission and Hydration

Water's role in neurotransmission is critical, as it underpins the brain's ability to communicate within itself and with the rest of the body:

- **Supporting Neurotransmitter Function**: The brain's neurotransmitters rely on proper hydration for their synthesis and function. These chemical messengers are responsible for transmitting signals across neurons, influencing everything from our movements to our thoughts and moods.
- **Mood Regulation**: Hydration has a direct impact on neurotransmitters like serotonin and dopamine, which regulate mood. Insufficient water intake can disrupt the balance and production of these neurotransmitters, leading to mood swings and challenges with emotional regulation.
- **Cognitive Effects**: Adequate hydration ensures smooth neurotransmission, which is essential for cognitive operations such as memory encoding, recall, and the capacity to learn new information. Dehydration

can cause cognitive fog, impacting these critical brain activities.

- **Energy Production**: Water is a key player in metabolic processes that provide energy to brain cells. Dehydration can impede these processes, leading to a reduction in energy available for cognitive functions and potentially resulting in mental fatigue and decreased alertness.

Ensuring ample water intake is thus crucial for the maintenance of neurotransmitter balance and activity, which, in turn, is vital for cognitive functioning, emotional stability, and overall brain health.

Detoxification and Hydration

The brain's ability to detoxify itself is profoundly supported by adequate hydration:

- **Glymphatic System Efficiency**: The glymphatic system is the brain's unique method of waste removal, operating primarily during sleep. This system depends on cerebrospinal fluid—largely composed of water—to clear out neural waste. Adequate hydration enhances the glymphatic system's ability to remove toxins, including proteins like beta-amyloid, which, if accumulated, are associated with Alzheimer's disease.
- **Preventing Neurodegenerative Diseases**: By aiding the glymphatic system, proper hydration may contribute to lowering the risk of neurodegenerative diseases. Efficient detoxification processes facilitated by

water intake can help prevent the buildup of harmful substances that can lead to cognitive decline.

- **Enhancing Blood Flow**: Hydration is key for maintaining blood flow to the brain, which is essential for delivering nutrients and removing waste. Dehydration can lead to reduced cerebral blood flow, impacting the brain's detoxification processes and overall function.
- **Supporting Brain Health and Longevity**: Chronic dehydration may have long-term detrimental effects on brain health. In contrast, regular and ample water intake supports brain function and, possibly, its longevity, contributing to better cognitive health over a lifetime.

Given the importance of hydration in facilitating the brain's detoxification processes, ensuring a regular intake of water is a simple yet effective strategy for maintaining cognitive health and potentially delaying the onset of age-related neurological diseases.

Sleep, Mood, and Stress Management Through Hydration

Hydration plays a vital role in regulating sleep, mood, and stress, all of which are essential for cognitive and emotional well-being:

- **Sleep Enhancement**: Adequate hydration contributes to better sleep quality. Dehydration can affect the natural balance of minerals and disrupt sleep patterns, leading to insomnia or unrestful sleep. Proper hydration helps maintain this balance, promoting restorative sleep essential for brain recovery and memory consolidation.

- **Mood Improvement**: Sufficient water intake can positively impact mood. Dehydration has been linked to increased incidences of mood disorders. Hydrating helps balance brain chemicals, like serotonin, that influence our emotional state, leading to a more stable and positive mood.
- **Stress Reduction**: Chronic dehydration can lead to elevated cortisol levels, the stress hormone, heightening feelings of anxiety. By staying hydrated, we can better manage physiological stress responses, maintaining calm and reducing the psychological impact of stress.
- **Reducing Anxiety**: Proper hydration can mitigate the physical symptoms of anxiety, such as a racing heart or tension, by ensuring smooth neurotransmission and overall nervous system health.
- **Cognitive and Emotional Resilience**: Consistent hydration helps the brain cope with the effects of stress, bolstering cognitive and emotional resilience. A hydrated brain can better adapt to stressful situations, maintaining focus and decision-making abilities.

By keeping the brain well-hydrated, we can help ensure that it functions at its best not only in terms of cognitive processes but also in managing the emotional and psychological challenges of everyday life.

Promoting Brain Health and Longevity with Hydration

Proper hydration is crucial for brain health over the lifespan and may contribute to neurological longevity:

- **Cellular Health**: Water is vital for maintaining the health of brain cells. Adequate hydration helps ensure that cells function properly and maintain their integrity, which is essential for all brain activities.
- **Cognitive Preservation**: Chronic dehydration can impact cognitive function over time. By staying well-hydrated, individuals can support their cognitive processes, potentially reducing the risk of age-related cognitive decline.
- **Neuroprotection**: Adequate water intake supports neuroprotective mechanisms, which can safeguard the brain against damage from environmental stresses and reduce the likelihood of developing neurodegenerative diseases.
- **Brain Metabolism**: Water is a key component in the brain's metabolic processes. Proper hydration ensures that the brain has the necessary resources to perform its complex functions efficiently, which is crucial for maintaining brain health as we age.
- **Cerebral Circulation**: Hydration has a direct impact on blood circulation within the brain. Sufficient hydration supports healthy blood flow, ensuring that

the brain receives the oxygen and nutrients it needs while removing metabolic waste.

Ensuring a consistent intake of water throughout one's life is an actionable and significant step toward enhancing brain health and promoting neurological vitality well into older age. Hydration stands as a foundational pillar for cognitive longevity, supporting the brain's structure, function, and protective mechanisms against the natural processes of aging.

Key Takeaways:

1. **Essential for Cellular Integrity**: Adequate hydration is essential for maintaining the size, shape, and function of brain cells, ensuring the integrity of neural connections vital for brain activity.
2. **Supports Cognitive Function**: Regular hydration facilitates optimal cognitive performance, reducing the risk of dehydration-induced impairments in memory, concentration, and decision-making.
3. **Neuroprotective Benefits**: Proper hydration contributes to the brain's self-maintenance and protective mechanisms, potentially guarding against neurodegenerative diseases.
4. **Crucial for Metabolic Processes**: Water is a key player in the brain's metabolism, necessary for energy production and the synthesis of critical molecules.
5. **Aids in Detoxification**: Hydration enhances the glymphatic system's efficiency in removing waste

products from the brain, crucial for preventing the buildup of harmful proteins.

6. **Improves Blood Flow**: Sufficient water intake is critical for maintaining cerebral blood flow, which is essential for the delivery of nutrients and oxygen to the brain.
7. **Promotes Longevity**: Hydration is believed to play a role in promoting neurological longevity, supporting cognitive health, and maintaining brain function as we age.

Introduction to Water and Weight Loss

Water, often heralded as the cornerstone of life, extends its bounty into the realm of weight management and health. Beyond its essential role in sustaining life and nurturing bodily functions, water emerges as a potent ally in the quest for weight loss. Let's look at the multifaceted role of water in promoting weight loss, unveiling its capabilities to suppress appetite, enhance metabolism, and support the body's digestive and detoxification systems. By understanding how to harness the power of water, individuals can unlock a natural, effective tool in achieving their weight loss goals, all while enhancing their overall health and vitality.

Appetite Suppression and Caloric Control

One of the most direct ways water influences weight loss is through its ability to modulate appetite and control caloric intake. Drinking water before meals can lead to a significant reduction in the number of calories consumed. This phenomenon can be attributed to water's capacity to fill the stomach, thereby inducing a feeling of fullness sooner during the eating process. A study highlighted in the chapter shows that participants who drank water before meals experienced a reduction in calorie consumption, contributing to a 44% greater weight loss compared to those who did not incorporate water into their pre-meal routine.

Furthermore, distinguishing between hunger and thirst signals plays a crucial role in caloric control. Often, the body's signals for thirst can be misinterpreted as hunger, leading individuals to consume food when, in reality, a glass of water would suffice. By staying adequately hydrated, individuals can more accurately interpret their body's needs, reducing unnecessary caloric intake and aiding in weight management.

Metabolism Enhancement

Water's influence extends into the realm of metabolism, the body's engine for burning calories. Research suggests that drinking water can temporarily boost the metabolic rate, an effect known as water-induced thermogenesis. A study cited in the chapter found that consuming 500ml of water increased the metabolic rate by 30% among both men and women, with the effect lasting up to 40 minutes after consumption. This metabolic acceleration contributes to the body's enhanced ability to burn calories, even when at rest, providing a supportive mechanism in the reduction of body weight.

The precise mechanisms behind water-induced thermogenesis are still under investigation, but the implications for weight loss are clear. By incorporating adequate water intake, individuals can support their body's metabolic processes, increasing energy expenditure and contributing to a caloric deficit essential for weight loss. This section underscores the importance of hydration not only for its direct health benefits but also for its role in enhancing metabolic efficiency and supporting weight reduction efforts.

These initial sections of the chapter lay the groundwork for understanding water's pivotal role in weight loss. Through appetite suppression and metabolic enhancement, water serves as a simple yet powerful tool in managing caloric intake and expenditure, essential components of a successful weight loss strategy.

Nutrient Absorption and Digestion

Water is integral to the body's digestive process, facilitating the breakdown of food and the absorption of nutrients. Adequate hydration ensures that the digestive system functions smoothly, preventing issues such as constipation, which can lead to bloating and discomfort. By aiding the transportation of nutrients throughout the body, water ensures that vital minerals and vitamins are effectively delivered to the cells that need them, supporting overall health and well-being.

Furthermore, water plays a crucial role in maintaining a healthy balance of gut bacteria, essential for not only digestion but also for metabolic health. Studies have shown that a well-hydrated body can more efficiently process food, absorb nutrients, and eliminate wastes, contributing to a more active metabolism and aiding weight loss efforts. The emphasis on hydration as a key element in digestive health highlights the interconnectedness of bodily systems and underscores the importance of water in maintaining a healthy weight and optimizing digestion.

Performance during Exercise

Hydration significantly impacts physical performance and endurance during exercise, a critical component of any weight loss program. Adequate water intake before, during, and after exercise ensures optimal performance, enabling individuals to exercise longer and at higher intensities. When the body is well-hydrated, it can efficiently regulate temperature through sweating, maintain blood volume, and reduce the risk of muscle cramps and fatigue. This not only enhances the immediate effectiveness of the workout but also aids in long-term fitness and weight loss goals.

Research supports the link between hydration and exercise performance, with dehydration shown to impair endurance, decrease strength, and reduce motivation. For those aiming to lose weight, ensuring proper hydration can make workouts more effective and enjoyable, leading to a greater calorie burn and improved muscle synthesis. This section of the chapter stresses the importance of viewing water intake as an essential part of the exercise regimen, emphasizing that hydration can significantly affect one's ability to engage in and benefit from physical activity.

In these sections, the narrative shifts to explore how water supports the body's digestive processes and enhances exercise performance, two pivotal aspects of a successful weight loss journey. By ensuring adequate hydration, individuals can optimize nutrient absorption, improve digestion, and maximize their physical performance, all of which contribute to effective weight management and overall health.

Detoxification

By facilitating the elimination of waste products and toxins through urine, sweat, and feces, adequate hydration ensures the body's detoxifying organs function optimally. This natural detoxification process supports a healthy metabolism, which is essential for effective weight management. The kidneys, liver, and digestive system rely on sufficient water intake to process and flush out toxins that, if accumulated, can adversely affect metabolic rates and the body's ability to burn fat.

Moreover, the process of burning fat releases toxins stored in fat cells into the bloodstream. Adequate water intake helps dilute these toxins and promotes their excretion, preventing potential reabsorption. A well-hydrated body is more efficient at processing and removing fats and toxins, contributing to a cleaner internal environment and supporting weight loss efforts.

Regulation of Body Functions

The human body comprises approximately 60% water, underscoring its vital role in nearly every bodily function, including those critical to weight loss and maintenance. Adequate hydration is essential for the nervous system, enabling neurotransmission and supporting brain functions that regulate appetite and satiety signals. It also plays a key role in the circulatory system, facilitating the efficient distribution of nutrients and oxygen to cells for energy production and metabolism.

Water's impact extends to the digestive system, where it aids in the breakdown of food and the absorption of nutrients, and to the excretory system, by supporting the elimination of waste products. Proper hydration ensures these systems work harmoniously, maintaining energy levels and optimizing bodily functions conducive to weight management. This section showcases how water is not just a passive component of the body but an active participant in regulating and supporting the systems that directly influence energy balance, metabolism, and ultimately, weight loss.

Body Weight Components

Overview of Body Weight Composition: Body weight is comprised of various components, each playing a critical role in overall health and functioning. These components include:

- **Water:** Constituting about 50-65% of the body, water is vital for every cell and organ, facilitating numerous biological processes.

- **Fat:** Fat or adipose tissue is essential for energy storage, hormone regulation, and insulation. While necessary, excessive fat, especially around organs, can pose health risks.
- **Muscle:** Muscle mass accounts for about 30-40% of body weight and includes skeletal, smooth, and water within muscles. Muscles burn calories even at rest, contributing to metabolism.
- **Bones:** Bones make up around 15% of an individual's total body weight, varying by age, sex, and density. They provide structure and support.
- **Other Components:** This includes organs (brain, liver, heart), blood, and other body fluids, each contributing to overall weight and health.

Factors that Influence Body Weight

Several factors can impact body weight, including:

- **Genetics:** Genetic makeup influences fat storage, distribution, and metabolic efficiency.
- **Diet and Exercise:** Caloric intake and physical activity levels are direct influencers of weight.
- **Environment:** Accessibility to healthy food and spaces for exercise, along with socio-economic factors, affect weight.
- **Psychological Factors:** Stress, anxiety, and sleep patterns can influence eating habits and weight.

- **Health Conditions and Medications:** Certain conditions and medications can lead to weight gain as a side effect.
- **Age:** Hormonal changes and muscle mass reduction can decrease metabolic rate over time.
- **Gender:** Hormonal differences affect muscle mass and fat distribution between men and women.
- **Sleep:** Quality sleep is essential for regulating hormones that control appetite and weight.

Role of Water in Metabolism and Energy Expenditure

Water is integral to metabolic processes and energy production. It helps maintain the structure of cells, assists in nutrient transport, and facilitates the removal of waste products. Adequate hydration can boost metabolism, as evidenced by studies showing that drinking 500ml of water can increase metabolic rate by 30% temporarily.

Effect of Water on Appetite and Satiety

Drinking water before meals has been shown to reduce hunger and caloric intake. Studies indicate that consuming water 30 minutes before eating can lead to decreased calorie consumption and contribute to weight loss. This effect is partly because water can be mistaken for hunger, so hydration may prevent unnecessary eating.

The Impact of Water Intake on Fat Loss vs. Muscle Loss

Hydration plays a crucial role in maintaining muscle mass and facilitating fat loss. Water aids in nutrient delivery to muscles, supports metabolic processes, and ensures effective workout recovery. While direct studies on water intake's effect on the fat-to-muscle loss ratio are limited, hydration's role in metabolism and muscle function suggests an indirect benefit.

Case Studies Demonstrating the Effect of Drinking Water on Weight Loss

Several case studies, such as those published in "Obesity" and by Virginia Tech, demonstrate that drinking water before meals leads to significant weight loss. Participants who consumed water before eating lost more weight than those who did not, highlighting water's role in weight management.

Overview of Scientific Studies

Research on water-induced thermogenesis, satiety, and hydration's effect on physical performance indicates positive effects on weight management. However, the calorie-burning effect of water-induced thermogenesis is relatively minor, and more comprehensive lifestyle changes are necessary for significant weight loss.

Water as Part of a Healthy Weight Loss Program

Water is a key element in weight loss strategies, aiding ketogenic diets, intermittent fasting, and calorie counting by promoting hydration, reducing appetite, and substituting for high-calorie drinks. Proper hydration is essential for these diets' effectiveness and overall health.

How to Properly Hydrate for Weight Loss

To incorporate hydration into a weight loss plan, set daily water intake goals, start the day with water, replace sugary drinks with water, and drink before meals to reduce appetite. Monitoring urine color can help ensure adequate hydration.

Key Takeaways:

1. **Appetite Suppression:** Drinking water before meals can reduce overall caloric intake by creating a feeling of fullness, thereby aiding in weight loss efforts.
2. **Boosts Metabolism:** Adequate hydration can enhance metabolic rate temporarily, facilitating increased energy expenditure even when at rest.
3. **Essential for Nutrient Absorption:** Water aids in the efficient breakdown and absorption of nutrients, which is vital for maintaining metabolic health and supporting weight loss.
4. **Improves Exercise Performance:** Staying hydrated is crucial for optimizing physical performance during exercise, allowing for longer, more intense workouts

that can burn more calories and contribute to weight loss.

5. **Supports Detoxification:** Regular water intake helps in flushing out toxins and waste products from the body, ensuring that metabolic processes are not hindered by their buildup.
6. **Integral to Body Function:** Water makes up a significant portion of the body and is essential for the proper functioning of all systems, including those directly and indirectly related to weight management.
7. **Influences on Body Composition:** Proper hydration helps maintain muscle mass and supports fat loss, showcasing the indirect effects of water intake on body composition during weight loss endeavors.
8. **Evidenced by Case Studies:** Research and case studies highlight the effective role of water consumption in achieving weight loss, underscoring the practical benefits of integrating water into a weight management plan.
9. **Scientific Support:** Although the calorie-burning impact of water-induced thermogenesis is relatively small, the collective evidence supports water's role in promoting satiety and enhancing metabolism.
10. **Inclusion in Diet Plans:** Water is a cornerstone of popular weight loss strategies, such as the ketogenic diet, intermittent fasting, and calorie counting, due to its

ability to support metabolic health and reduce unnecessary caloric intake.

11. **Hydration Strategies for Weight Loss:** Setting daily intake goals, substituting water for sugary beverages, and drinking water before meals are practical steps to leverage hydration for weight management.
12. **Awareness of Overhydration Risks:** While hydration is key, it's also important to avoid the dangers of overhydration, which can lead to electrolyte imbalances and health issues.

The Miracle Molecule and Our Aging Body

Our bodies undergo numerous changes as we journey from infancy through to old age, with one of the most fundamental yet overlooked aspects being the fluctuation in our body's water content. This journey begins with a newborn, whose body is comprised of approximately 78% water, and culminates in the elderly, where the body's water content may decrease to about 50-55%. This dynamic shift in hydration levels is not just a mere curiosity of human biology; it reflects the profound biological and physiological demands placed on our bodies at different life stages. Understanding these changes is crucial for optimizing our health, as it allows us to adjust our hydration needs to match our body's evolving requirements, thereby supporting vital functions and overall well-being.

The Newborn Hydration Phenomenon

The high water content in newborns, which stands at about 78%, is primarily intracellular and is concentrated within the muscle tissues. This significant percentage is essential for supporting the rapid growth and development that characterize the earliest stages of life. In infants, the high metabolic rate and the need for rapid cell proliferation make water an indispensable resource. Water serves as the medium for numerous biochemical reactions, aids in the transport of nutrients, facilitates waste elimination, and helps regulate body temperature. The infant's dependency on a high level of hydration underscores the critical role of water in sustaining life from its very inception.

Transitioning Through Childhood and Adolescence

As children transition from infancy through childhood and into adolescence, there is a notable reduction in their total body water percentage, which stabilizes at approximately 60-65% by the age of one. This level generally remains constant throughout the childhood and teenage years. This reduction is directly linked to the body's developmental changes, specifically the increased development of bone and muscle tissue. As the body composition shifts to accommodate more solid tissues, the relative proportion of body water naturally diminishes. This change illustrates the body's remarkable ability to adapt its water content in response to its growing and changing structure.

Water Content in Adulthood

In adulthood, the body's water content finds a new norm, typically constituting 50-60% of an individual's body weight. This range is influenced by various factors including sex, body composition, and overall health status. Men, for instance, tend to have a higher percentage of body water compared to women, attributed to their greater muscle mass. Muscle tissues, known for their higher water content relative to fat, contribute significantly to this difference. However, as we advance in age, there is a gradual decline in muscle mass, and consequently, a reduction in the body's water content. This gradual decrease highlights the ongoing changes in hydration needs as adults age, emphasizing the importance of adapting our water intake to maintain optimal health.

Understanding these stages of hydration throughout life not only sheds light on the physiological intricacies of our bodies but also underscores the importance of tailoring our hydration practices to suit our changing needs. From the water-rich beginnings of infancy to the more conservative hydration state of old age, our body's journey through water content changes is a testament to its adaptability and the pivotal role of water in sustaining life.

Aging and Dehydration

As individuals progress into their senior years, the percentage of body water continues to decline, potentially reaching as low as 45-50%. This decrease in body water content is attributed to a natural loss of muscle mass and decreased efficiency in kidney function. Furthermore, older adults often experience a reduced sense of thirst, which significantly contributes to inadequate fluid intake. The repercussions of dehydration in the elderly are severe and wide-ranging, including urinary tract infections (UTIs), pneumonia, confusion, and even falls. These health implications highlight the critical need for heightened awareness and proactive measures to ensure adequate hydration in older adults.

Factors Leading to Increased Risk of Dehydration in Aging

Several factors exacerbate the risk of dehydration as one ages. The decline in kidney function with age means that the body becomes less capable of conserving water when dehydrated. Additionally, the diminished sense of thirst reduces the natural inclination to drink water, further complicating hydration efforts. Certain medications and medical conditions, such as diabetes, which prompts frequent urination, can increase the risk of dehydration. Older adults are also more susceptible to heat-related issues, like heatstroke, which can rapidly lead to severe dehydration.

Health Implications of Dehydration in Older Adults

Dehydration in older adults can manifest through various symptoms, including confusion, weakness, and exhaustion. It can also lead to more severe conditions such as urinary tract infections and, in the absence of appropriate intervention, escalate to heat exhaustion, heat stroke, and in extreme cases, death. The susceptibility to dehydration coupled with these potential outcomes underscores the necessity of recognizing and addressing hydration needs promptly.

Preventive Measures Against Dehydration

Preventing dehydration in older adults involves a multifaceted approach focused on ensuring regular fluid intake. This is particularly crucial during hot weather or periods of physical exertion. Older adults are encouraged to consume a variety of hydrating fluids, including water, low-fat milk, and 100% fruit juice. Incorporating foods with high water content, such as watermelon, cucumbers, and strawberries, into the diet can also contribute to overall hydration. It is advisable to limit or avoid beverages that can lead to further dehydration, such as those containing caffeine or alcohol, due to their diuretic effects.

Ensuring that older adults maintain adequate hydration is not merely a measure to prevent discomfort but a vital component of preserving health and preventing serious, potentially fatal, health issues. Encouraging regular fluid intake, alongside a diet rich in water-dense foods and mindful of diuretic beverages, can significantly mitigate the risks associated with dehydration in the aging population.

Key Takeaways:

1. **Dynamic Water Content:** The human body undergoes significant changes in water content from infancy through old age, starting at about 78% water in newborns and potentially declining to 45-50% in seniors.
2. **Infant Hydration Needs:** Newborns and infants require a high percentage of water in their bodies to support rapid growth, development, and the high metabolic rate characteristic of early life stages.
3. **Childhood and Adolescence Transition:** During these growth periods, the body's water percentage naturally decreases to about 60-65% as bone and muscle tissue develop, reducing the relative proportion of body water.
4. **Adult Water Content:** In adults, body water constitutes 50-60% of body weight, influenced by factors such as sex, body composition, and overall health. Men typically have a higher percentage of body water than women due to greater muscle mass.
5. **Aging and Dehydration Risks:** Elderly individuals face increased risks of dehydration due to factors like reduced kidney efficiency, decreased muscle mass, and a diminished sense of thirst, emphasizing the importance of adequate fluid intake.

6. **Health Implications of Dehydration**: Dehydration in older adults can lead to severe health issues, including UTIs, pneumonia, confusion, and even life-threatening conditions like heatstroke.
7. **Preventive Measures**: It's crucial for older adults to regularly consume fluids, particularly in hot weather or when exerting physically. Hydration sources should include water, low-fat milk, and 100% fruit juice, alongside a diet rich in foods with high water content. Avoiding caffeine and alcohol, which can exacerbate dehydration, is also recommended.

The Dangers of Dehydration

Water is the lifeline of every cell, tissue, and organ in our bodies, ensuring they function optimally. Yet, the significance of hydration is often overlooked until the body begins to suffer from the lack of it. Dehydration, even in its mildest form, can trigger a plethora of health issues ranging from headaches and fatigue to severe dizziness. This chapter delves into the negative impacts of dehydration, providing insights on how to recognize the signs of needing more water and the vital role water plays in our overall health and well-being.

Dehydration occurs when the body loses more fluids than it takes in, leading to an imbalance that affects the body's ability to carry out normal functions. Some signs and symptoms of dehydration include dry mouth, tiredness, thirst, decreased urine output, dark yellow urine, dry skin, headache, and dizziness. The effects of dehydration on the body are profound, impacting everything from physical performance to cognitive function. Common causes include not drinking enough water, excessive sweating, diarrhea, and vomiting. Preventing dehydration is key, involving adequate daily water intake, monitoring fluid loss, and adjusting water consumption based on activity levels and environmental conditions.

SIGNS: Recognizing Dehydration

Recognizing dehydration early is crucial for prompt intervention. Signs that you might not be drinking enough water include feelings of lethargy, unexplained hunger, dryness in the mouth, skin, and eyes, excessive thirst, dark-colored urine, disorientation, and headaches. It's vital to note that dehydration can develop quickly, within just a few hours without water, escalating from mild to severe and requiring urgent medical attention.

Physical Performance and Hydration

For athletes and individuals engaged in any form of physical activity, hydration is non-negotiable. Dehydration can severely hamper an athlete's performance, affecting endurance, strength, and coordination, and can lead to dangerous conditions like heat stroke. The American College of Sports Medicine advises drinking about 16-20 ounces of water four hours before exercise and rehydrating post-exercise based on the intensity and duration to counteract fluid loss and optimize performance.

Comprehensive Effects of Dehydration

Dehydration's grip extends beyond mere physical performance, affecting cognitive functions, digestive health, kidney performance, skin condition, and cardiovascular health. From impairing brain function and leading to constipation to promoting kidney issues and causing skin problems, dehydration disrupts the body's harmony. Maintaining hydration is essential for the prevention and management of these issues, highlighting water's indispensable role in health and disease prevention.

The Body's Alert System for Hydration

Our bodies have an innate system to signal hydration needs, with thirst being a primary indicator. However, by the time you feel thirsty, your body is already experiencing dehydration. Recognizing this and other preemptive signs of dehydration can prevent the adverse effects associated with water deficiency. Responding promptly to these signals by increasing fluid intake is crucial for maintaining optimal health.

Ten Signs to Tell if You are Dehydrated

Dehydration can manifest through various signs, from dark yellow urine and a dry, sticky mouth to fatigue, feverish skin, irritability, and a reduced attention span. Recognizing these signs can prevent the escalation of dehydration to more severe health issues. It's also important to understand that certain conditions, like diabetes, and medications can increase dehydration risk, necessitating increased fluid intake.

Preventive Measures Against Dehydration

Staying ahead of dehydration involves more than just responding to thirst. It requires a proactive approach to fluid intake, incorporating water and other hydrating fluids into your daily routine, especially before, during, and after physical exertion. Eating water-rich foods and avoiding diuretics like caffeine and alcohol can also support hydration. Understanding and responding to the body's hydration cues are essential for preventing dehydration and maintaining health.

Key Takeaways:

1. Proper hydration is essential for health, but needs vary widely among individuals.
2. Water intake should be adjusted based on activity level, climate, health status, and physiological cues.
3. Recognizing the signs of dehydration is crucial for maintaining optimal hydration.
4. Regular monitoring and adjustment of water intake can help prevent dehydration and its associated health risks.

HYDRATION

Water is fundamental to life, however, there isn't a one-size-fits-all answer to how much water an individual needs. Factors such as age, gender, activity level, and climate can significantly influence our hydration requirements.

1. Understanding Hydration Needs

The body's need for water varies greatly among individuals and is influenced by several key factors. Age and gender play crucial roles, with adults typically needing more water than children, and men generally requiring more than women. Activity level is another critical factor; individuals who engage in regular exercise or physical labor lose more water through sweat and hence have higher hydration needs. Additionally, living in hot or dry climates can increase the body's demand for water to cool down and maintain a normal temperature. Recognizing these factors is the first step towards personalized hydration.

2. The Role of Beverages in Hydration

While water is the best and most direct source of hydration, other beverages like tea, coffee, and soda also contribute to our daily water intake. However, it's essential to approach these alternatives with caution. Sugary drinks, for example, can lead to dehydration and contribute to inflammatory conditions, negatively impacting joint health. The key is balancing these beverages with plain water to ensure optimal hydration without the adverse effects of excess sugar or caffeine.

3. Daily Water Intake Recommendations

Guidelines from the National Academies of Sciences suggest that men aged 19 and older consume 3.7 liters (about 16 cups) of water per day from all beverages and foods, and women consume 2.7 liters (about 11 cups). However, these are general recommendations that serve as a starting point. Individual needs may vary based on the factors discussed earlier, highlighting the importance of tailoring water intake to one's specific circumstances.

4. Recognizing Dehydration and Its Signs

Dehydration can manifest through various signs, such as unexplained fatigue, persistent hunger pangs, dryness of the mouth, skin, and eyes, excessive thirst, darkly colored urine, disorientation, and headaches. Understanding these signals can help prevent mild dehydration from escalating into severe dehydration, which can have more serious health implications.

5. Hydration and Physical Activity

For individuals engaging in physical activity, proper hydration is crucial for maintaining performance and preventing heat-related illnesses. The American Council on Exercise suggests specific guidelines for hydrating before, during, and after workouts to offset fluid loss through sweating and support recovery. Additionally, incorporating electrolytes into post-exercise hydration can help replenish what's lost through sweat, especially after prolonged or intense sessions.

6. When to Drink Water for Optimal Hydration

Hydrating first thing in the morning kickstarts the body's internal systems and supports the flushing out of toxins. It's also advisable to avoid caffeine on an empty stomach due to its potential for increasing stomach acidity. Drinking a glass of water before bed can aid in overnight recovery and detoxification processes. Following these timing guidelines can help optimize hydration and its benefits.

7. Factors Influencing Water Needs

Exercise intensity, environmental conditions, personal health status, and dietary choices all play roles in determining an individual's hydration needs. Being attentive to the body's signals, such as thirst and the color and volume of urine, can provide valuable cues for adjusting water intake. It's also worth noting that high-fiber diets, caffeine, and alcohol consumption can increase the body's water requirements.

Tap Water: Your Everyday Source

Tap water is the most accessible and commonly used source of water for many households. It comes from local municipal supplies and undergoes treatment processes to remove harmful contaminants and pathogens, making it safe for consumption. The quality and taste of tap water can vary significantly depending on the region, influenced by the source of the water and the treatment methods employed. For those concerned about specific contaminants or the overall quality of their tap water, home water testing kits are available. These kits can help identify any potential issues, ensuring that your tap water is safe for drinking.

Exploring Other Water Types

- **Spring Water**: Sourced directly from natural springs, this type of water is valued for its purity and mineral content. Spring water is filtered naturally through the earth and bottled at the source, preserving its natural minerals and unique taste. However, consumers should look for quality certifications to ensure the water meets safety standards.
- **Purified Water**: This category includes water from any source, including tap, spring, or ground water, that has been purified to remove impurities and contaminants. The purification process can involve methods like reverse osmosis, distillation, or deionization, resulting in water that is virtually free of dissolved substances.
- **Mineral Water**: Known for its content of various minerals like calcium, magnesium, and potassium, mineral water comes from mineral springs and is bottled directly from the source. These minerals can offer health benefits and contribute to the water's taste.
- **Distilled Water**: Produced by boiling water and then condensing the steam back into liquid, distilled water is free from impurities and minerals. Its lack of minerals gives it a flat taste, making it less preferred by some for drinking.
- **Filtered Water**: Involves treating tap or well water with various filtration systems to remove chlorine, lead, and other contaminants. Filtration can significantly improve

the taste and safety of water, making it a popular choice for drinking and cooking.

Safety First: Ensuring Your Water is Clean

Ensuring the cleanliness and safety of your drinking water, regardless of the source, is paramount. For homeowners using tap or well water, investing in a high-quality water filtration system can be a wise decision. These systems can remove a wide range of contaminants, improving both the safety and taste of the water. Bottled water consumers should choose brands with a proven track record of quality testing and environmental stewardship. Regular testing of well water is also advisable to detect any contaminants that could pose health risks.

Beyond Water: Hydration Alternatives

Hydration is not limited to water alone. Fruits and vegetables with high water content, such as cucumbers, watermelons, and oranges, can also contribute to your daily fluid intake. Herbal teas and broths offer additional hydration options, providing both fluids and essential nutrients. Diversifying your sources of hydration can make meeting your daily fluid needs more enjoyable and nutritious.

Environmental Considerations

The environmental impact of bottled water, particularly plastic bottles, is a growing concern. These bottles contribute to resource depletion, pollution, and landfill waste. Opting for reusable water bottles and home filtration systems can significantly reduce this impact, offering a more sustainable way to stay hydrated.

The Verdict

Selecting the best source of water comes down to individual needs and preferences, considering factors like safety, taste, and environmental impact. Staying informed about your local water quality and available alternatives can help you make choices that align with your health goals and environmental values. Remember, staying adequately hydrated is crucial for overall health, so prioritize finding hydration solutions that work for you.

Key Takeaways:

1. **Tap Water Accessibility**: Tap water is widely available and typically safe for consumption thanks to local treatment processes. However, its quality can vary, making it essential to test your water if you have specific concerns.
2. **Variety of Water Sources**: Beyond tap water, there are several options including spring, purified, mineral, distilled, and filtered water. Each type offers different benefits in terms of taste, mineral content, and purity.
3. **Safety and Cleanliness**: Ensuring the water you drink is clean and safe is crucial, regardless of the source. Regular testing, especially for well water, and considering a home filtration system can enhance the safety and taste of your drinking water.

4. **Alternative Hydration Sources**: Hydration doesn't solely depend on drinking water. Foods with high water content, herbal teas, and broths also contribute to your daily fluid intake, offering nutritional benefits alongside hydration.
5. **Environmental Considerations**: The environmental impact of bottled water, especially in plastic containers, highlights the importance of considering sustainable hydration practices, such as using reusable bottles and tap water filtration systems.
6. **Personalized Hydration Needs**: The optimal source and amount of water depend on individual factors including age, activity level, climate, and health conditions. Listening to your body's signals, like thirst and observing the color of your urine, can help guide adequate daily water intake.
7. **Importance of Staying Informed**: Understanding local water quality, available water sources, and the environmental impact of your choices allows for informed decisions about hydration that support both health and sustainability.

Tips for Ways to Drink Water

It's not always easy to remember to drink water throughout the day.

To boost your daily water intake, consider these proven strategies and inventive methods:

1. Begin each day with water to kickstart hydration.
2. Always have a reusable water bottle handy.
3. Use reminders for regular water breaks.
4. Place a water bottle within easy reach at your workstation.
5. Enhance water's flavor with lemon, lime, or cucumber.
6. Consume water before meals to aid digestion.
7. Choose water over sugary beverages.

8. Equip your car with a water bottle for hydration on the move.
9. Maintain hydration during and post-exercise.
10. Swap a daily coffee or tea for water occasionally.
11. Enjoy herbal teas or fruit-infused water for variety.
12. Eat fruits and veggies high in water content, like watermelon and cucumber.
13. Track intake with a water app to ensure you're meeting your goals.
14. Drink water if you're feeling off—it might be thirst.
15. Have water accessible at your bedside for morning and evening sips.
16. Prefer gradual sipping over consuming large amounts at once.
17. Use waiting times as opportunities to hydrate.
18. Always fill your bottle before leaving home.
19. Opt for sparkling water to refresh without added sugar.
20. Minimize alcohol to avoid dehydration.
21. Set daily bottle-finishing goals.
22. Hydrate during TV time, including commercial breaks.
23. Store a pitcher in the fridge for chilled water.
24. Counteract tiredness with hydration—it could signal dehydration.
25. Encourage friends or colleagues to join in hydration challenges.
26. Include a water bottle in your gym or travel bag.
27. Combat airplane cabin dryness with extra water.

28. Choose soups and smoothies for their high water content.
29. Hydrate during work or study breaks.
30. Balance caffeinated drinks with water.
31. Drinking through a straw can increase your intake.
32. Keep a compact water bottle for convenience.
33. Hydrate if you wake up thirsty during the night.
34. Take water breaks in long meetings or seminars.
35. Order water with meals when dining out.
36. Refill from water fountains in public spaces.
37. Stress or anxiety? Water can help soothe nerves.
38. Celebrate reaching hourly hydration milestones.
39. If you often refill, consider a larger bottle.
40. Stay hydrated on hikes and outdoor adventures.
41. Alternate water and alcoholic drinks at social events.
42. Rehydrate post-hot baths or showers.
43. Improve tap water with a filter for better taste.
44. Integrate water consumption into your daily habits.
45. Record your intake to track progress.
46. Stay attentive to your thirst signals for optimal hydration.

Staying hydrated in hot weather is crucial for maintaining good health and preventing heat-related illnesses. Here are several ways to stay hydrated in the heat:

1. Drink plenty of water: This is the most obvious and important way to stay hydrated. Keep a water bottle

with you at all times and sip on it regularly throughout the day.

2. Electrolyte drinks: In addition to water, consider consuming electrolyte-rich beverages like sports drinks or coconut water. These drinks help replenish the electrolytes lost through sweating.
3. Eat hydrating foods: Include fruits and vegetables with high water content in your diet. Watermelon, cucumbers, oranges, and strawberries are excellent choices.
4. Avoid or limit alcohol and caffeine: Both alcohol and caffeine act as diuretics, which can increase fluid loss. If you do consume them, make sure to drink extra water to compensate.
5. Set reminders: It's easy to forget to drink enough water when you're busy or distracted. Use reminders on your phone or set specific times to drink water throughout the day.
6. Dress appropriately: Wear lightweight and breathable clothing that allows sweat to evaporate. This can help regulate your body temperature and prevent excessive fluid loss.
7. Take frequent breaks in shaded areas: If you're outdoors in the heat, try to find shaded areas to rest and cool down. This can help reduce your body's water loss through sweating.

8. Use a misting spray or wet towel: Spraying water mist on your face or using a wet towel on your neck or forehead can provide instant relief and help cool down your body.
9. Avoid intense physical activity during peak heat hours: If possible, schedule your outdoor activities during cooler parts of the day, such as early morning or late evening, to minimize fluid loss.
10. Monitor urine color: Pay attention to the color of your urine. If it's dark yellow, it's a sign that you need to drink more fluids. Aim for a pale, light yellow color, indicating proper hydration.

Eat Your Water

Understanding the Value of Water-Rich Foods: Integrating foods with high water content into your daily meals is a natural and efficient method to maintain hydration. These foods not only contribute significantly to your overall fluid intake but also come packed with essential nutrients that bolster health and vitality. This segment delves into the myriad advantages of embracing a diet abundant in water-rich foods and spotlights some prime examples of such hydrating nourishments.

Aiding Weight Management: Water-dense foods typically boast a lower calorie profile while offering a satiating feeling, making them allies in weight management endeavors. These foods can curb overeating tendencies and seamlessly fit into a health-conscious dietary routine, promoting a lean and nourished physique.

Skin Health Enhancer: Hydrated skin is synonymous with radiant and youthful skin. Foods rich in water content aid in flushing out toxins and encourage the regeneration of skin cells, culminating in a glowing and rejuvenated skin appearance. Items like watermelon, cucumbers, and strawberries are especially beneficial for enhancing skin health.

Digestive Harmony: A well-hydrated body ensures a smoothly operating digestive system, preventing constipation and facilitating efficient nutrient absorption. High water content foods, alongside being fiber-rich, contribute to digestive well-being and regularity.

Champion Hydrating Foods:

1. **Cucumbers**: At 96% water content, cucumbers top the list for hydrating foods. They are also a good source of fiber.
2. **Watermelon**: Known for its 92% water content, watermelon also provides vitamin C and lycopene.
3. **Strawberries**: Delicious and 91% water, strawberries are rich in antioxidants and vitamin C.
4. **Spinach**: This leafy green is 91% water and loaded with vitamins A and K.
5. **Broccoli**: With 90% water content, broccoli is also rich in fiber and vitamin C.
6. **Grapefruit**: Offering 88% water, grapefruit is a vitamin C powerhouse.

7. **Carrots**: At 87% water, carrots are a great source of vitamin A.
8. **Tomatoes**: Comprising 95% water, tomatoes are beneficial for heart health.
9. **Cantaloupe**: This melon is 90% water and a good source of vitamin C and beta-carotene.
10. **Pineapple**: With 87% water content, pineapple is known for its bromelain content, which aids digestion.

Incorporating these hydrating foods into your diet not only assists in meeting your daily water intake goals but also enriches your body with vital nutrients, promoting a healthier, well-hydrated you. While direct water consumption remains crucial, augmenting your hydration through a diet rich in water-laden foods offers a complementary path to maintaining your body's fluid balance, enhancing skin health, supporting weight management, and ensuring digestive health. Here are my families top recipes for eating your water, enjoy!

Appetizer

Papaya Salsa

Ingredients

- 1 papaya
- 1 lime juiced
- 1 habanero chile
- 2 avocados
- ½ cup red onion
- Cilantro, minced
- Salt and pepper to taste

Preparation

1. Combine 1 diced small papaya and the juice of 1 lime in a bowl. Mash 1/2 chopped seeded habanero chile and 1/2 teaspoon kosher salt into a paste with a large knife, then add 1/2 cup cilantro and mince. Add the chile mixture to the bowl along with 2 diced avocados and 1/2 diced red onion; stir until combined and season with salt.

Mango Salsa

Ingredients:

- 2 ripe mangoes, peeled and diced
- 1/2 red onion, diced
- 1 red bell pepper, diced
- 1 jalapeño pepper, seeded and minced
- 2 tablespoons chopped fresh cilantro leaves

- 2 tablespoons lime juice
- Salt and pepper, to taste

Preparation:

1. In a large bowl, combine mangoes, red onion, red bell pepper, jalapeño pepper, cilantro leaves, and lime juice.
2. Toss gently to combine.
3. Season with salt and pepper to taste.
4. Serve chilled.

Tomato and Basil Bruschetta

Ingredients:

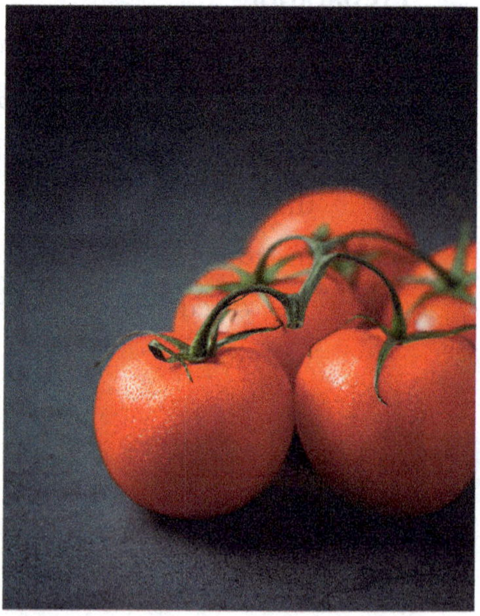

- 4 ripe tomatoes, diced
- 1/4 red onion, diced
- 2 cloves garlic, minced
- 1/4 cup chopped fresh basil
- 2 tablespoons balsamic vinegar
- Salt and pepper to taste
- Baguette, sliced and toasted

Preparation:

1. Combine diced tomatoes, red onion, garlic, basil, and balsamic vinegar in a large bowl.
2. Season with salt and pepper to taste.
3. Let the mixture sit for at least 10 minutes to allow the flavors to meld.
4. Serve the tomato mixture on top of toasted baguette slices.

Bell Pepper Salsa:

Ingredients:

- 2 cups chopped bell peppers (mixed colors)
- 1 cup cherry tomatoes, halved
- 1/4 cup red onion, chopped
- 1 jalapeño, seeded and minced
- 1/4 cup fresh cilantro, chopped
- 1 lime, juiced
- Salt and pepper, to taste

Preparation:

1. In a large bowl, combine bell peppers, tomatoes, red onion, jalapeno

Grilled Pineapple Salsa

Ingredients:

- 1 pineapple, peeled and cored

- 1 red bell pepper, diced
- 1/2 red onion, diced
- 1 jalapeno pepper, seeded and minced
- 1/4 cup chopped cilantro
- 2 tablespoons lime juice
- Salt and pepper to taste

Preparation:

1. Preheat grill to medium-high heat.
2. Cut pineapple into slices and grill for 3-4 minutes per side, until slightly charred.
3. Remove pineapple from grill and let cool.
4. Dice grilled pineapple and combine with red bell pepper, red onion, jalapeno pepper, cilantro, and lime juice in a large bowl.
5. Season with salt and pepper to taste.
6. Serve with tortilla chips or as a topping for grilled chicken or fish.

Baba Ghanoush

Ingredients

- 2 large eggplants
- 8 garlic cloves, minced
- 5 tablespoons tahini
- 5 tablespoons of fresh squeezed lemon juice (about 1 lemon)
- 2 tablespoons of olive oil

- Handful of chopped parsley
- 1 teaspoon sumac (optional, it is a Lebanese spice)

Preparation:

1. Preheat oven to 376 degrees F.
2. Bake the eggplants on a baking sheet for 30 minutes.
3. When cool to touch, slice eggplant in half, scoop out the flesh, and chop, then drain in a colander at least 10 minutes.
4. In a bowl, mix the minced garlic, tahini, and lemon juice with the eggplant to form a smooth paste. Add the olive oil, sprinkle with parsley and serve with crackers, pita chips, carrots, celery and/or cucumbers.

Salads

Watermelon Feta Salad

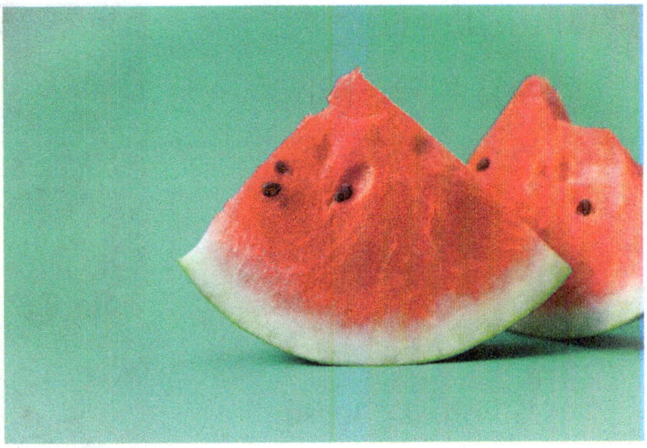

Ingredients:

- 1 small watermelon, cubed
- 1/2 cup crumbled feta cheese
- 1/4 cup thinly sliced red onion
- 1/4 cup chopped fresh mint leaves
- 1/4 cup chopped fresh parsley leaves
- Salt and pepper, to taste

Preparation:

1. In a large bowl, combine watermelon, feta cheese, red onion, mint leaves, and parsley leaves.
2. Toss gently to combine.
3. Season with salt and pepper to taste.
4. Serve chilled.

Strawberry and Spinach with Goat Cheese

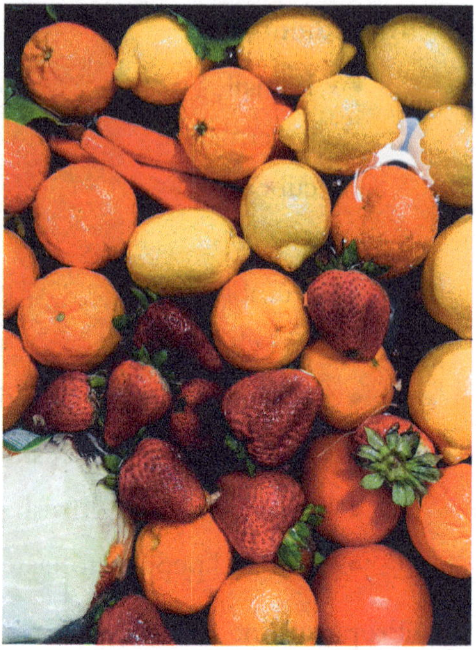

Ingredients

- 4 cups baby spinach
- 1 cup sliced strawberries
- 1/2 cup crumbled goat cheese
- 1/4 cup chopped pecans
- 2 tablespoons balsamic vinegar
- 2 tablespoons olive oil
- Salt and pepper to taste

Preparation:

1. Combine baby spinach, sliced strawberries, crumbled goat cheese, and chopped pecans in a large bowl.
2. In a separate bowl, whisk together balsamic vinegar, olive oil, salt, and pepper.
3. Drizzle the dressing over the salad and toss to combine.
4. Serve chilled.

Tomato Cucumber Salad

Ingredients:

- 2 medium cucumbers, sliced
- 2 medium tomatoes, chopped
- 1/4 red onion, thinly sliced
- 2 tablespoons chopped fresh parsley leaves
- 1 tablespoon olive oil
- 1 tablespoon red wine vinegar
- Salt and pepper, to taste

Preparation:

1. In a large bowl, combine cucumbers, tomatoes, red onion, and parsley leaves.
2. In a small bowl, whisk together olive oil, red wine vinegar, salt, and pepper.
3. Drizzle dressing over salad and toss to combine.
4. Serve chilled.

Bean Salad

Ingredients:

- 1 can of black beans
- 1 can of kidney beans
- 1 can of chickpeas

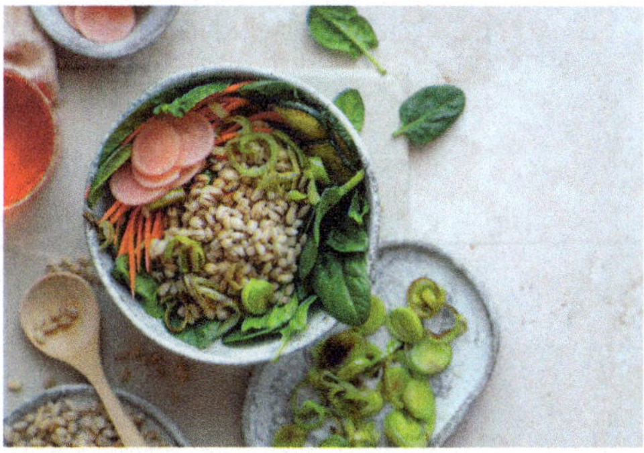

- 1 red bell pepper, chopped
- 1 green bell pepper, chopped
- 1 small red onion, chopped
- 1/4 cup of chopped fresh cilantro
- 1/4 cup of olive oil
- 2 tablespoons of red wine vinegar
- 1 tablespoon of honey
- 1 teaspoon of ground cumin
- Salt and pepper to taste

Preparation:

1. Rinse and drain the black beans, kidney beans, and chickpeas in a colander.
2. In a large bowl, combine the beans, chopped red and green bell peppers, and chopped red onion.
3. In a separate bowl, whisk together the olive oil, red wine vinegar, honey, cumin, salt, and pepper until well combined.
4. Pour the dressing over the bean mixture and stir well to combine.
5. Add in the chopped cilantro and stir again.
6. Cover the bowl with plastic wrap and refrigerate for at least 30 minutes to allow the flavors to meld together.
7. Serve the bean salad chilled, garnished with additional cilantro if desired.

Watermelon and Feta Salad

Ingredients:

- 1 small seedless watermelon
- 200g feta cheese
- 1/4 cup chopped fresh mint leaves
- 1/4 cup chopped fresh basil leaves
- 1/4 cup extra virgin olive oil
- 2 tbsp balsamic vinegar
- Salt and freshly ground black pepper to taste

Preparation:

1. Cut the watermelon into small cubes and place in a large bowl.
2. Cut the feta cheese into small cubes and add to the bowl with the watermelon.
3. Add the chopped mint and basil leaves to the bowl.
4. In a separate bowl, whisk together the olive oil and balsamic vinegar.
5. Pour the dressing over the watermelon and feta salad and toss gently to combine.
6. Season with salt and pepper to taste.
7. Serve chilled.

Celery, Apple, and Fennel Salad

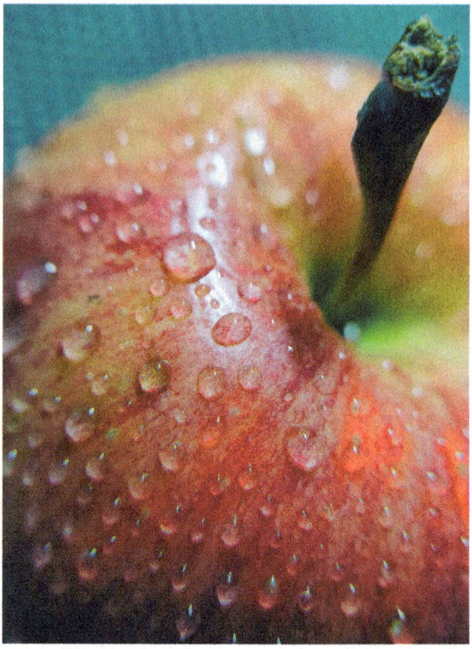

Ingredients:

- 4 cups celery, thinly sliced
- 2 apples, cored and thinly sliced
- 1 fennel bulb, thinly sliced
- 1/4 cup walnuts, chopped
- 1/4 cup fresh parsley, chopped
- 1/4 cup extra-virgin olive oil
- 2 tbsp fresh lemon juice
- Salt and pepper, to taste

Preparation:

1. In a large bowl, combine celery, apples, fennel, walnuts, and parsley.
2. In a small bowl, whisk together olive oil and lemon juice. Season with salt and pepper.
3. Pour the dressing over the salad and toss to combine.

Strawberry Spinach Salad with Poppy Seed Dressing

Ingredients:

- 6 cups fresh spinach
- 2 cups fresh strawberries, sliced
- 1/2 cup red onion, thinly sliced
- 1/2 cup almonds, slivered
- 1/3 cup extra-virgin olive oil
- 3 tbsp apple cider vinegar
- 2 tbsp honey
- 1 tbsp poppy seeds
- Salt and pepper, to taste

Preparation:

1. In a large bowl, combine spinach, strawberries, red onion, and almonds.
2. In a small bowl, whisk together olive oil, apple cider vinegar, honey, and poppy seeds. Season with salt and pepper.
3. Pour the dressing over the salad and toss to combine.

Cucumber Salad

Ingredients:

- 2 English cucumbers thinly sliced
- 1 teaspoon salt
- 1 red onion thinly sliced

- 1 cup distilled white vinegar
- 1/2 cup water
- 1/2 cup granulated sugar
- 2 tablespoons fresh dill minced

Preparation:

1. Season cucumbers with salt in a large bowl and let sweat 1 hour. Drain liquids and toss cucumbers with onion slices.
2. In a small saucepan over high heat, pour in white vinegar and water and stir in sugar until dissolved and liquid turns clear, 3 to 5 minutes.
3. Pour over cucumbers and onions. Stir in dill. Cover with plastic wrap and refrigerate 1 hour. Serve cold or at room temperature.

Mediterranean Cucumber Salad

Ingredients:

- 2 English cucumbers, diced
- 1 cup cherry tomatoes, halved
- 1 cup chickpeas (rinsed)
- ¼ cup finely sliced red onion
- ½ cup crumbled feta cheese
- 1 tablespoon chopped fresh dill
- 1 tablespoon chopped fresh parsley
- 1 tablespoon chopped fresh mint

- 2 tablespoons fresh lemon juice
- ¼ cup olive oil
- Sea salt, to taste

Preparation:

1. Begin by gathering and prepping all of your ingredients according to the ingredient list above to have ready and organized for use.
2. Place the diced cucumbers, the cherry tomatoes, the chickpeas, the red onion, ¼ cup of the feta cheese, half of the dill, half of the parsley and half of the mint into a large bowl; add the lemon juice and the olive oil, along with a couple of good pinches of sea salt, and gently toss together to combine.
3. Spoon the salad out onto a serving platter or into a salad bowl, and sprinkle over top the remaining ¼ cup of feta cheese and the remaining herbs, and serve.

Fresh Tomato Salad

Ingredients

- 2 pints grape tomatoes halved, or 3 cups chopped tomatoes
- ¼ cup red onion thinly sliced
- 1 tablespoon of fresh basil
- 1 tablespoon of fresh parsley
- 1 tablespoon of fresh dill
- 1 teaspoon dried oregano

Dressing

- 3 tablespoons olive oil
- 1 tablespoon balsamic vinegar
- Salt and pepper to taste

Preparation:

1. Place tomatoes, red onion, in a shallow bowl.
2. Drizzle with olive oil and vinegar. Toss to combine.
3. Season with salt, pepper, and fresh herbs to taste.

Italian Tomato Salad

Ingredients:

- ½ cup chopped red onion (about ½ small red onion)
- 1 pint (12 ounces or 2 cups) cherry tomatoes, halved
- 1 pound additional tomatoes (about 1 large, 2 medium or 3 small), cut into bite-sized wedges
- ¼ cup thinly sliced fresh basil and/or small basil leaves (or substitute parsley, dill and/or chives)
- 1 cup lettuce, ripped into bite size pieces
- Option to add your favorite cheese, mozzarella or feta taste great
- 2 tablespoons extra-virgin olive oil
- 2 tablespoons balsamic vinegar
- ½ teaspoon salt, to taste
- Freshly ground black pepper, to taste

Preparation:

1. To assemble the salad, spread the tomato wedges over a large serving platter. Layer about one-third of the onions on top. Add half of the cherry tomatoes, followed by a layer of any optional additions, followed by another one-third of the onions. Finish with the remaining cherry tomatoes, followed by the remaining onions, and sprinkle the basil all over.
2. Drizzle the olive oil over the salad, followed by the balsamic vinegar. Sprinkle the salt and several twists of black pepper on top.

Radish Salad

Ingredients:

- 1 large head of romaine lettuce
- 4 small cucumbers (or 1 English cucumber) - thinly sliced
- 10-11 radishes (1 bunch) - trimmed and thinly sliced
- 1/2 cup fresh chives (1 bunch) - finely chopped

Lemon Vinaigrette

- 3 tablespoons extra virgin olive oil
- 1 tablespoon freshly squeezed lemon juice
- zest from 1/2 lemon – optional
- salt and pepper to taste

Preparation:

1. Make the vinaigrette. In a small bowl, combine and stir together 3 tbsp extra virgin olive oil, 1 tbsp freshly squeezed lemon juice, 1/2 tsp salt and 1/8 tsp ground black pepper. Set aside.
2. Rinse and paper towel pat dry all vegetables.
3. Combine 4 small thinly sliced cucumbers, 1 bunch thinly sliced radishes and 1/2 cup finely chopped fresh chives.
4. Chop 1 large romaine lettuce into bite-sized pieces and add it to the salad.
5. Drizzle with lemon vinaigrette and toss gently until salad is evenly coated. You can also drizzle without tossing the salad and serve.

Broccoli Cauliflower Salad

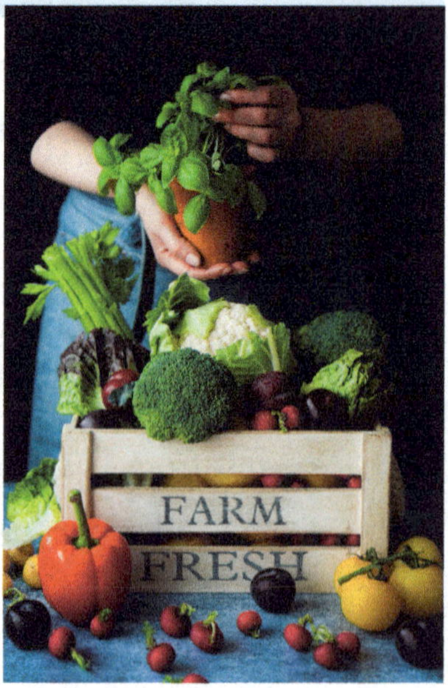

Ingredients:

- 4 small cucumbers
- 2 small broccoli heads
- 1 medium cauliflower head
- 1 bunch fresh radishes (11-12 radishes)
- 1/4 cup fresh green onions, chopped

- 1/4 cup fresh dill, chopped (or 1 bunch)
- 1/2 cup (120g) mayonnaise
- 1/2 cup (120g) plain Greek yogurt
- Salt and pepper to taste

Preparation:

1. Wash all vegetables and pat dry. Cut broccoli into small florets.
2. Remove and discard cauliflower core and cut the rest into small florets.
3. Thinly slice halved cucumbers and radishes. Finely chop green onions and fresh dill. Add to the salad.
4. In a small bowl, stir together 1/2 cup mayo, 1/2 cup plain Greek yogurt and 1 teaspoon fine salt. Add dressing to the salad and toss well to combine, just before serving.

Vegetable Salad

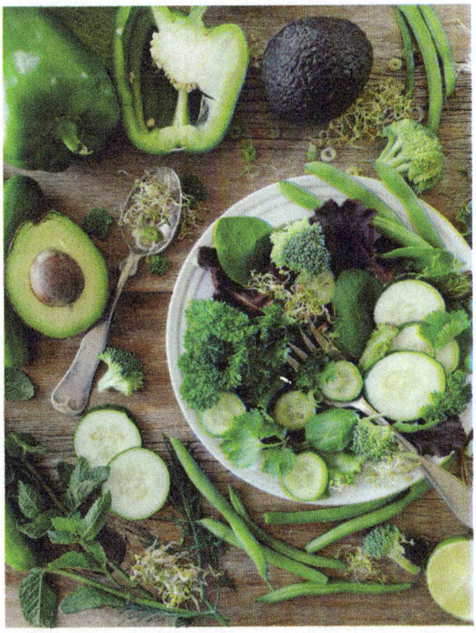

Ingredients:

- 1 cup red cabbage – shredded
- 1 large yellow bell pepper
- 10 oz yellow/red cherry tomatoes
- 1 large orange bell pepper

- 1 large red bell pepper
- 5 green onions
- 1 English cucumber
- 1 medium carrot
- 10 parsley stems (1/2 cup)
- 1 pack dill (0.66 oz)

Dressing

- 4 tablespoons sunflower oil
- 2 tablespoons white wine vinegar
- 1 teaspoon table salt or to taste
- ¼ teaspoon ground black pepper or to taste
- 2 cloves garlic – pressed (more ok if garlic eater)

Preparation:

1. Into a large bowl, shred 1 cup red cabbage.
2. Cut large yellow bell pepper into 8 wedges
3. Repeat for large orange bell pepper and red bell pepper.
4. Cut 1 English cucumber into half, then into quarter and slice.
5. Peel, wash, paper towel pat dry and grate 1 medium carrot.
6. Halve red/yellow cherry tomatoes.
7. Chop green onions and parsley stems (about 1/2 cup) and finely chop dill.
8. Gently mix all vegetables.

Dressing:

In a small bowl, combine 4 tbsps sunflower oil, 2 tbsps white wine vinegar, 1 tsp table salt, 1/4 tsp ground black pepper and peel/press 2 garlic cloves into the liquid. Whisk the dressing and pour over the salad. Gently stir in the dressing into the salad just until mixed in. Refrigerate the salad for at least 2 hours to give it time to absorb the dressing.

Cabbage, Carrot, Cucumber Salad

Ingredients:

- Green cabbage, medium (2 lb) – shredded
- English cucumber
- Orange bell pepper
- Carrot
- Fresh green onions (5-6 stems)
- Fresh dill (about 1/2 cup chopped)

Dressing

- Extra virgin olive oil
- Red wine vinegar
- 1 tsp. monk fruit sugar
- Salt and pepper to taste

Preparation:

1. Wash and paper towel pat dry your veggies.
2. Into a large bowl, thinly shred cabbage.
3. Slice cucumber into the bowl with cabbage.

4. Cut 1 orange bell pepper into quarter, remove the seeds and slice.
5. Grate carrot.
6. Finely chop 1 bunch green onions and 1 bunch dill; add the herbs to the salad.

Make the Dressing.

In a small bowl, combine and whisk 1/2 cup grapeseed oil, 1/4 cup red wine vinegar, 1 tbsp sugar and 1 tsp fine salt. Let it sit for 5-10 mins in order for sugar and salt to dissolve a bit. Pour the dressing over the salad and give the salad a good stir in order for dressing to fully cover all the veggies. Refrigerate salad for at least 2 hours before serving. Stir, taste and add salt if necessary before serving.

Honey Marinated Grapefruit

Ingredients:

- 4 ruby red grapefruit
- 2 tablespoon honey
- 1 tablespoon fresh mint, chopped

Preparation:

1. Squeeze the juice of 1 grapefruit and grate 1 tsp of zest, set aside.
2. Warm the honey in the microwave for 15 seconds. Add the juice and zest and mix well.
3. Peel the remaining grapefruit and segment into pieces.
4. Arrange on a plate and cover with the marinade.

5. Sprinkle with chopped mint.

Citrus Fruit Salad

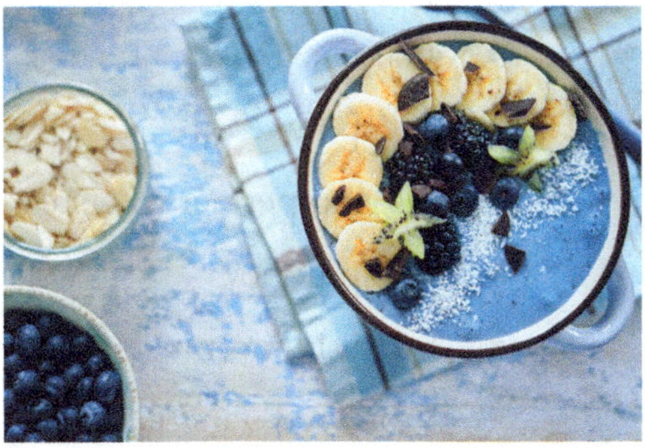

Ingredients:

- 3 large handfuls of mixed lettuce leaves, (swiss chard, spinach, kale)
- 2 tablespoons chopped parsley leaves
- 1 tablespoon chopped cilantro leaves
- 1 tablespoons sunflower seeds
- 1 ruby red grapefruit
- 1 tablespoon olive oil
- 1 tablespoon fresh lemon juice
- 1 tablespoon fresh orange juice

Preparation

1. Put the lettuce leaves, parsley, cilantro and sunflower seeds into a bowl.
2. Cut the grapefruit into segments and add to the bowl.
3. Drizzle the olive oil and citrus juices over the salad.

Roasted Radish and Carrot Salad

Ingredients:

- 1 bunch of radishes
- 4 large carrots
- 2 tbsp olive oil
- Salt and pepper to taste
- 1 tbsp honey
- 1 tbsp Dijon mustard
- 2 tbsp red wine vinegar
- 1/4 cup chopped fresh parsley
- 1/4 cup crumbled feta cheese

Preparation:

1. Preheat oven to 400°F (200°C).
2. Trim the tops and bottoms of the radishes and carrots, and slice them into thin rounds.
3. Toss the sliced radishes and carrots with olive oil, salt, and pepper on a baking sheet. Roast in the preheated oven for 20-25 minutes, until the vegetables are tender and lightly browned.
4. While the vegetables are roasting, make the dressing. In a small bowl, whisk together honey, Dijon mustard, red wine vinegar, and salt and pepper to taste.
5. Once the vegetables are done, transfer them to a large bowl and let them cool slightly.

6. Add the dressing and chopped parsley to the bowl and toss everything together until the vegetables are coated in the dressing.
7. Serve the salad warm or at room temperature, topped with crumbled feta cheese.

Watercress Salad

Ingredients:

- 3 tablespoons white wine or champagne vinegar
- 1/2 teaspoon Dijon mustard
- 3/4 teaspoon
- 3 tablespoons extra-virgin olive oil
- Salt and pepper to taste

For the salad:

- 1/3 cup whole almonds
- 1 teaspoon olive oil
- 1/2 small red onion
- 1/2 cup cold water
- 6 ounces watercress (about 2 bunches)
- 1 medium Granny Smith apple
- 2 ounces shaved Pecorino Romano cheese (about 2/3 cup)

Preparation:

1. Make the dressing. Place 3 tablespoons white wine or champagne vinegar, 1/2 teaspoon Dijon mustard, 3/4 teaspoon kosher salt, and a few grinds freshly ground black pepper in a small bowl. Whisk until the salt is dissolved. While whisking constantly, slowly drizzle in 3 tablespoons extra-virgin olive oil and continue whisking until emulsified.
2. Place 1/3 cups almonds, 1 teaspoon olive oil, and 1/4 teaspoon kosher salt in a medium skillet over medium heat. Cook, stirring constantly, until the almonds darken in color slightly and are very fragrant, 6 to 8 minutes. Immediately transfer to a paper towel-lined plate. Let cool while you prepare the onion.
3. Thinly slice 1/2 small red onion. Place in a small bowl, cover with 1/2 cup cold water, and set aside for 10 minutes to make the onion less potent. Coarsely chop the almonds.
4. Thinly slice 1/2 small red onion. Place in a small bowl, cover with 1/2 cup cold water, and set aside for 10 minutes to make the onion less potent. Coarsely chop the almonds.
5. Drain the onion and add to the bowl. Top with the almonds. Drizzle half the dressing over the salad and gently toss to coat. Add more dressing if desired (you may have some left over). Serve immediately.

Watercress, Apple and Pear Salad

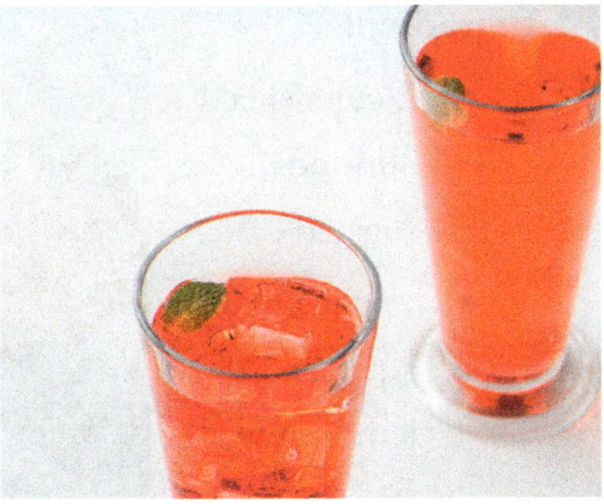

Ingredients:

- 3 cups watercress
- 1 green apple
- 1 pear
- ⅓ cup almonds

Salad Dressing

- 2 tbsp olive oil
- ½ lemon , juiced
- 1 tsp brown mustard
- 1 tbsp honey
- 1 tsp mayonnaise
- Salt and pepper to taste

Preparation:

1. Wash and trim watercress.
2. Slice apple and pear into matchsticks. Place in a bowl of salted cold water to stop oxidation.
3. Toast almonds in a dry pan over medium heat for 1-2 minutes. Remove from the pan and roughly chop.

Salad Dressing

1. Mix together in a mason jar, olive oil, lemon juice, seeded mustard, honey, mayonnaise and salt. Shake well.

Lemony Kale Salad

Ingredients:

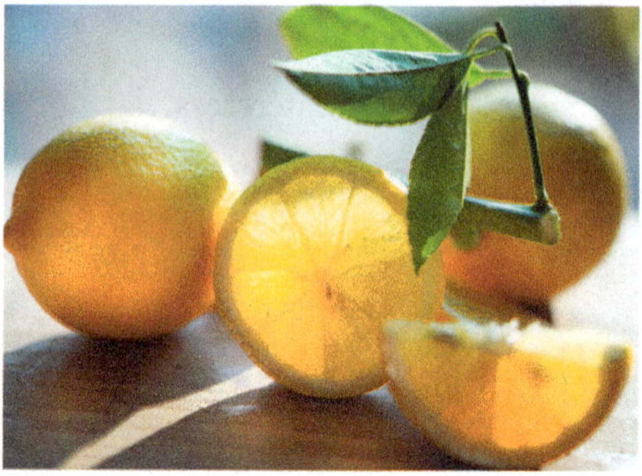

- 2 cups sliced almonds, toasted
- ⅓ cup freshly squeezed lemon juice (from 2 to 4 lemons)
- 1 1/4 cups extra-virgin olive oil + 2 T for bread crumbs
- 6 cloves garlic, minced
- 10 to 12 ounces washed and dried kale leaves, thick stems removed (weight after trimming)
- 1½ cups freshly grated Parmesan
- Salt and pepper to taste
- Touch of cayenne pepper (optional)
- 1 cup diced bread crumbs, day old French bread works well

Preparation:

2. Toast almonds on a skillet until golden brown and fragrant. Remove from pan and set aside to cool.
3. Toast bread crumbs in skillet with 2 tablespoons of olive oil,

4. In a bowl, combine lemon juice and 1 heaping teaspoon salt. Slowly whisk in olive oil. Add garlic cloves and set aside to steep.
5. Working in batches, cut the kale into thin ribbons: gather a large handful of leaves, bunch together tightly, and use the other hand to slice into ¼-inch-thick pieces. the idea is to end up with a kind of slaw.
6. f starting with a bunch of curly kale, wash, dry, and remove leaves from stem.
7. Finely chop kale leaves and add to a medium-large bowl.
8. Whisk together dressing ingredients and drizzle a teeny bit (around 1/2 tsp) onto the kale leaves.
9. Massage dressing into kale leaves until the leaves darken in color and become tender and silky.
10. Toss with remaining dressing and top with freshly grated parmesan cheese.
11. Place croutons in a plastic bag or between two paper towels. Crush into small pieces to sprinkle over the kale salad.

Place chopped kale in a very large bowl. Sprinkle surface with almonds and then with cheese, if using. Remove and discard garlic cloves from dressing. Pour half the dressing over the salad and toss. Taste for dressing and salt and add more as needed, tossing to coat thoroughly. Serve within 1 hour.

Bok Choy Salad

Ingredients:

Dressing

- 1/4 cup light brown sugar
- 1/4 cup olive oil
- 2 tablespoons red wine vinegar
- 1 tablespoon soy sauce

For the salad:

- 2 tablespoons olive oil
- 1 package ramen noodles crumbled, seasoning packet discarded
- 1/4 cup sliced almonds
- 1 bunch baby Bok choy sliced about 5 – 6 bulbs
- 5 scallions chopped

Preparation:

1. To make the dressing, in a small bowl, whisk together brown sugar, olive oil, vinegar, and soy sauce. Allow flavors to blend at room temperature while preparing the rest of the salad.
2. In a large sauce pan over medium heat, heat olive oil until shimmering. Reduce heat to low. Add ramen noodles and almonds; sauté until toasted, about 10 minutes, stirring frequently to avoid scorching.

3. In a large bowl, combine baby Bok choy, scallions, and crunchy mix. Drizzle salad dressing over the top and toss until uniformly combined.

Broccoli Salad

Ingredients;

- 5 cups broccoli cut into bite-sized pieces
- 2 cups cauliflower cut into bite-size pieces
- ½ cup shredded red cabbage
- 1 yellow bell pepper, sliced thinly
- 2 carrots, sliced thinly
- ⅓ cup red onion diced
- ½ cup dried cranberries
- ¼ cup sunflower seeds
- ½ cup bacon bits

Dressing

- 1 cup mayonnaise
- 5 tablespoons apple cider vinegar
- 2 tablespoons of monk fruit sugar (granulated can do the job as well)
- Salt and pepper to taste

Preparation:

1. Whisk together dressing ingredients in a medium bowl. Set aside.

2. In a large bowl, combine broccoli, carrots, cabbage, onion, cranberries, sunflower seeds, and bacon bits. Pour the prepared dressing over and mix well.
3. Refrigerate for at least one hour before serving.

Okra and Tomato Salad

Ingredients:

- 1 pound fresh okra, cut into 1/2-inch pieces
- 1 15-ounce can of black beans, drained and rinsed
- 1 ear of corn (fresh sweet peak-season corn preferred)
- 1 large, white onion, diced
- 1 pound (about 15-20) cherry tomatoes, halved
- 3 tablespoons extra virgin olive oil
- 1 avocado, sliced
- Salt and pepper to taste

Preparation:

1. In a large pot of salted boiling water, blanch the okra until it's bright green, about 30 seconds. Drain well and allow to cool to room temperature. Cut the okra into 1/2 inch pieces, and discard the stems.
2. Add the okra, beans, corn, onion, olive oil, sea salt, and pepper to a large mixing bowl, and toss gently until the olive oil is evenly distributed. Chill for 30 minutes or more. Before serving, cut the avocado into 1/4-inch pieces and gently toss with the salad. Add more salt and pepper to taste if necessary.

Spinach and Strawberry Salad

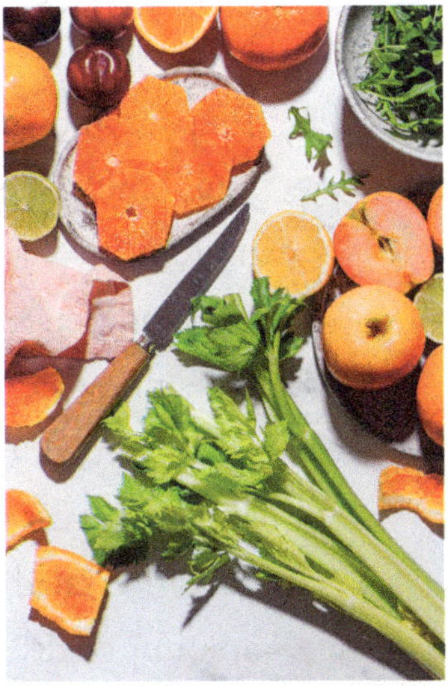

Ingredients

- 3/4 cup raw pecans
- 1/2 small red onion very thinly sliced
- 10 ounces fresh baby spinach
- 1 quart strawberries hulled and quartered (about 1 pound)
- 3/4 cup crumbled feta cheese

Poppy seed Dressing:

- 1/4 cup balsamic vinegar
- 3 tablespoons extra-virgin olive oil
- 1 1/2 tablespoons poppy seeds
- 1 1/2 tablespoons honey
- 1/2 teaspoon Dijon mustard
- Salt and pepper to taste

Preparation:

1. Toast the pecans: Preheat the oven to 350 degrees F. Spread the pecans in a single layer on an ungreased baking sheet. Bake for 8 to 10 minutes, until the pecans smell fragrant and the center of a pecan is tan when the pecan is broken in half.

2. Place the sliced onions in a bowl and cover with cold water. Let sit while you prepare the rest of the salad (this keeps their flavor but removes the harsh onion bite).
3. Prepare the dressing: In small mixing bowl or large liquid measuring cup, whisk together all of the dressing ingredients—vinegar, oil, poppy seeds, honey, mustard, salt, and pepper—until well combined.
4. Assemble the salad: Place the spinach in a great big serving bowl. Add the strawberries. Drain the red onion and add it as well. Drizzle about half of the dressing over the salad and toss to coat the leaves. Assess the amount of dressing. You want the spinach leaves to be nicely moistened but not swimming in dressing. Add the feta and pecans. Toss lightly to combine. Serve immediately, with extra dressing on the side as desired.

Celery, Apple and Parmesan Salad

Ingredients:

- 8 celery ribs plus ½ cup celery leaves
- 1 red apple
- 1 tablespoon white wine vinegar
- ½ tablespoon Dijon mustard
- 1 teaspoon maple syrup or sugar
- ½ teaspoon salt
- 3 tablespoons olive oil
- ¼ cup shaved Parmesan cheese

Preparation:

1. Thinly slice the celery ribs. Measure out the celery leaves. Thinly slice the red apple.
2. In a medium bowl, whisk together the white wine vinegar, Dijon mustard, maple syrup or sugar, and salt. Gradually whisk in the olive oil one tablespoon at a time.
3. In another bowl, toss together the celery and celery leaves with the apple, dressing, and Parmesan cheese shavings. Serve immediately or refrigerate until serving. This tastes best the day of making, but you can refrigerate leftovers for a few days (refresh them with a little vinegar or salt if necessary).

Cabbage, Apple and Celery Coleslaw

Ingredients:

- 1/2 head green cabbage (about 4 cups)
- 1/2 head red cabbage (about 4 cups)
- 3 stalks celery
- 1 thinly sliced apple
- 1 small red onion (about ½ cup)
- 2 tablespoons rice vinegar
- 2 tablespoons cider vinegar
- ¼ teaspoon dill
- 4 tablespoons olive oil
- Salt and pepper to taste

Preparation:

1. Thinly slice the cabbage and measure out 8 cups. Thinly slice the onion and the celery.
2. In a medium bowl, whisk together the rice vinegar, cider vinegar, dill, chili powder, and salt. Whisk in the olive oil tablespoon by tablespoon until a creamy emulsion forms.
3. In a large bowl, toss the cabbage, red onion, and celery with the dressing. Add ground black pepper to taste, and additional salt as necessary. Serve immediately. (Note: The slaw is best served the day that it is made; leftovers do not save well. One idea is to only add dressing to the vegetables that you plan to eat.)

Classic Waldorf Salad

Ingredients:

- 5 celery ribs, trimmed and chopped
- 2 apples, chopped
- Grapes, any color and as much or little as you like, (I use about ½ cup sliced)
- 1 scallion, trimmed and chopped
- ¼ cup walnuts, chopped
- 2 tablespoons mayonnaise
- 2 tablespoons of plain non-fat yogurt
- ½ teaspoon celery seeds
- Salt and pepper to taste

- Handful of romaine lettuce (optional)

Preparation:

1. Put the celery, apples, grapes, scallions, and walnuts in a large bowl.
2. Make the dressing: Put mayonnaise, yogurt, celery seeds and salt and pepper into a small bowl and whisk.
3. Add dressing to salad, give it a good toss and serve.

Cucumber and Mint Salad

Ingredients:

- 4 tablespoons of chopped mint leaves
- 1 large cucumber, chopped
- 2 celery ribs, trimmed and chopped
- 2 teaspoons champagne vinegar (or white wine vinegar0
- ½ cup plain, non-fat yogurt

Preparation:

1. Mix together the chopped mint, cucumber an celery in a serving bowl.
2. In a smaller bowl, whisk the vinegar into the yogurt.
3. Pour dressing over the salad and serve.

Watermelon Salad

Ingredients:

- 4 cups cubed watermelon
- 1 cup crumbled feta cheese

- 1/2 cup fresh mint leaves, chopped
- 1/4 cup red onion, thinly sliced
- 2 tbsp olive oil
- 1 tbsp balsamic vinegar
- Salt and pepper, to taste

Preparation:

1. In a large bowl, combine watermelon, feta cheese, mint leaves, and red onion.
2. In a small bowl, whisk together olive oil, balsamic vinegar, salt, and pepper.
3. Pour the dressing over the watermelon mixture and gently toss to combine.

Tomato Basil Quinoa Salad:

Ingredients:

- 2 cups cooked quinoa
- 2 cups cherry tomatoes, halved
- 1/4 cup fresh basil leaves, chopped
- 1/4 cup red onion, chopped
- 1/4 cup crumbled feta cheese
- 2 tbsp olive oil
- 1 tbsp balsamic vinegar
- Salt and pepper, to taste

Preparation:

1. In a large bowl, combine quinoa, tomatoes, basil, red onion, and feta cheese.
2. In a small bowl, whisk together olive oil, balsamic vinegar, salt, and pepper.
3. Pour the dressing over the quinoa mixture and toss to combine.

Celery and Apple Salad:

Ingredients:

- 4 cups chopped celery
- 2 apples, cored and thinly sliced
- 1/2 cup chopped walnuts
- 1/2 cup plain Greek yogurt
- 2 tbsp honey
- 1 tbsp lemon juice
- Salt and pepper, to taste

Preparation:

1. In a large bowl, combine celery, apples, and walnuts.
2. In a small bowl, whisk together Greek yogurt, honey, lemon juice, salt, and pepper.
3. Pour the dressing over the celery mixture and toss to combine.

Farmer's Market Salad

This recipe came from one of my favorite farmer's at my local market. Thank you Josh!

Ingredients:

- 6 ounces baby spinach leaves
- 1 cucumber, chopped
- 8 radishes, trimmed and thinly sliced
- 2 carrots, peeled and thinly sliced
- 1 scallion, trimmed and chopped
- 2 tablespoons chopped parsley leaves
- 2 tablespoons of olive oil
- 1 lime juiced

Preparation:

1. Combine the vegetables and parsley in a large bowl.
2. Pout the olive oil and lime juice over and toss well.

Avocado and Grapefruit Salad

Ingredients:

- 3 tablespoons of olive oil
- 1 teaspoon honey
- 1 small red onion chopped
- 1 teaspoon Dijon mustard
- 4 avocados, pitted, peeled and slice

- 1 ruby red grapefruit (any color will do), peeled and segmented
- 1 cup of arugula

Preparation:

1. In a small bowl mix whisk the oil, honey, onion and mustard together.
2. Add the avocados, grapefruit and arugula, toss well with the dressing.

Tuscany Tomato Panzanella

Ingredients:

- 5 oz or ½ loaf of a rustic Italian bread (I used Ciabatta) cut into 1-inch cubes
- Extra Virgin Olive oil
- Kosher salt
- 2 ¼ lb ripe tomatoes I used vine ripe tomatoes, cut into small wedges or cubes
- ¼ cup red wine vinegar
- 2 garlic cloves minced
- ½ teaspoon Dijon mustard
- 1 teaspoon fesh thyme optional
- Black pepper
- 2 Small shallots peeled and thinly sliced
- ½ cup packed fresh basil torn

- 4 oz fresh baby mozzarella optional (more to your liking)

Preparation:

1. Heat the oven to 400 degrees F.
2. In a large mixing bowl, combine bread cubes with large drizzle of extra virgin olive oil and a generous pinch of kosher salt. Toss to make sure the bread is well coated (save the bowl for later use). Spread the bread cubes on a sheet pan and bake in heated oven for about 10 minutes or until golden (the edges should get crisp, while the bread gains some color and crisp but remains still a bit chewy).
3. Place a large colander over the same mixing bowl. Place the tomatoes in the colander and sprinkle with kosher salt. Toss briefly with your hand. Set aside for a few minutes to allow the tomatoes to release their juices in the mixing bowl.
4. When ready, move the colander with the tomatoes to the sink for now, and use the mixing bowl with the tomato juice to make the dressing. Add red wine, ½ cup extra virgin olive oil, garlic cloves, Dijon mustard, thyme, and a large pinch of black pepper. Whisk to combine.
5. Add the tomatoes, bread cubes, shallots, basil and mozzarella (if using) to the mixing bowl and toss to coat with the dressing. Allow the salad to sit for 20 to 30 minutes before serving.

6. Give the salad a gentle toss and transfer to a serving platter. Garnish with a few more fresh basil leaves, if you like.

Capri Watermelon and Basil Salad

Ingredients:

- 8 cups cubed ripe seedless watermelon (1 8-pound watermelon)
- 2 organic mini cucumbers or ½ English cucumber (1 cup sliced)
- 2 ounces Feta cheese crumbles
- Zest of 1/2 lemon
- 4 basil leaves
- Salt to taste

Preparation:

1. Chop the watermelon into cubes. Slice the cucumber into coins.
2. Arrange the watermelon and cucumbers on a platter. Sprinkle with feta crumbles, lemon zest, and sea salt. Taste and adjust flavors as desired. (If you'd like, you can add freshly ground black pepper or a drizzle of olive oil.) Serve immediately. If making ahead, refrigerate the cubed watermelon separately: it releases a lot of water after it is cut. Then assemble the salad directly before serving.

Kale Salad with Currants and Pecorino

Ingredients:

- 1 bunch of kale, stems discarded and leaves cut crosswise into ribbons
- ½ cup shaved pecorino cheese
- 3 tablespoons of olive oil
- 1 tablespoon squeezed lemon juice
- Salt and pepper to taste
- 1/3 cup pine nuts
- ¼ cup currants
- 3 medium radishes, thinly sliced
- ½ green pepper, thinly sliced
- ¼ cup chopped mint leaves

Preparation:

1. Preheat oven to 350 degrees F.
2. In a large bowl, toss kale with ¾ of the pecorino, plus the olive oil and lemon juice, season with salt and pepper. Let stand for 10 minutes to tenderize the kale. You can massage the kale to help tenderize the leaves.
3. Meanwhile, place the pine nuts in a metal pan, toast in the oven for 5 minutes until slightly browned. Transfer to a bowl, let cool.
4. Just before serving, sprinkle pine nuts, currants, radishes, green pepper, and mint over kale, and toss. Serve with remaining pecorino.

Salad on a Stick

Ingredients:

- 6 ounces creamy feta cheese, cut into 10 to 12 cubes
- ½ English cucumber, halved lengthwise, then sliced into half moons
- 1 small green pepper, cored, cut into 10 to 12 square pieces
- 10 to 12 cherry or grape tomatoes
- 10 to 12 pitted Kalamata olives

Dressing

- 1 garlic clove, minced
- ½ lime, juice of
- 1 tablespoon red wine vinegar
- 1 tablespoon olive oil
- Kosher salt and black pepper
- 1 tsp dried oregano

Preparation:

1. Prepare 10 to 12 small bamboo skewers (I used 6-inch skewers). Take one skewer and thread through it one feta cube, a slice of cucumber, a piece of green pepper, one cherry tomato, and, lastly, one kalamata olives at the very top. Repeat till you have 10 to 12 small skewers of feta and veggies.
2. In a small bowl, add the garlic, lime juice, and red wine vinegar. Season with kosher salt, black pepper and the

dried oregano. Whisk together, and as you do, drizzle the extra virgin olive oil and keep whisking.

3. Arrange the skewers on a serving platter and pour the dressing over. Serve or refrigerate for later.

Fruit Salad

Ingredients:

- ⅔ cup fresh orange juice
- ⅓ cup fresh lemon juice
- ⅓ cup packed brown sugar
- ½ teaspoon grated orange zest
- ½ teaspoon grated lemon zest
- 1 teaspoon vanilla extract
- 2 cups cubed fresh pineapple
- 2 cups strawberries, hulled and sliced
- 3 kiwi fruit, peeled and sliced
- 3 bananas, sliced
- 2 oranges, peeled and sectioned
- 1 cup seedless grapes
- 2 cups of blueberries

Preparation:

1. Bring orange juice, lemon juice, brown sugar, orange zest, and lemon zest to a boil in a saucepan over medium-high heat. Reduce heat to medium-low, and simmer until slightly thickened, about 5 minutes.

Remove from heat, and stir in vanilla extract. Set aside to cool.

2. Layer the fruit in a large, clear glass bowl in this order: pineapple, strawberries, kiwi fruit, bananas, oranges, grapes, and blueberries. Pour the cooled sauce over the fruit. Cover and refrigerate for 3 to 4 hours before serving.

SOUP

Bone broth is a nutritious and flavorful base for soups, stews, or enjoyed on its own as a warming drink. Rich in minerals and collagen, making your own bone broth at home is surprisingly simple and a great way to utilize leftover bones from meals. Here's how to make a basic bone broth:

Ingredients:

- 2-3 pounds of mixed bones (chicken, beef, pork, or fish), preferably from grass-fed or organically raised animals
- 2 medium carrots, roughly chopped
- 2 celery stalks, roughly chopped
- 1 large onion, quartered (no need to peel)
- 4 garlic cloves, smashed (optional)
- 2 bay leaves
- A few sprigs of fresh thyme or 1 teaspoon dried thyme
- 1 teaspoon whole black peppercorns
- 2 tablespoons apple cider vinegar
- Water to cover (about 12 cups)
- Salt to taste

Instructions:

1. **Prep the Bones:** If you're using raw bones, especially beef or pork, roasting them first will add depth of flavor. Preheat your oven to 400°F (200°C), place the bones on a baking sheet, and roast for 30 minutes.

2. **Combine Ingredients:** Place the roasted (or raw, if using chicken or fish bones) bones in a large stockpot. Add the carrots, celery, onion, garlic (if using), bay leaves, thyme, peppercorns, and apple cider vinegar. Cover with water so that the bones are submerged by 2 inches.
3. **Slow Cook:** Bring the mixture to a gentle boil over medium-high heat. Reduce the heat to low, allowing the broth to simmer gently. For chicken or fish bones, simmer for at least 8-24 hours; for beef or pork bones, aim for 24-48 hours. The longer you simmer, the more flavorful and nutritious your broth will be.
4. **Skim the Fat:** Throughout the cooking process, skim off any foam and fat that rises to the surface with a spoon or ladle.
5. **Strain the Broth:** After simmering, remove the pot from heat. Use a fine-mesh sieve to strain the broth into a large container, discarding the solids.
6. **Season:** Taste the broth and add salt as needed. Remember, the flavor should be rich and savory, but not overly salty.
7. **Cool and Store:** Allow the broth to cool to room temperature before transferring it to the refrigerator. Once cool, a layer of fat will harden on the surface, which you can remove if desired.
8. **Store or Freeze:** Keep the broth in the refrigerator for up to 5 days, or freeze it in smaller portions for up to 3

months. Ice cube trays are great for freezing small, usable portions.

Bone broth can be enjoyed on its own, seasoned with a little salt, pepper, and herbs. It's also a versatile ingredient in a myriad of dishes, from soups and stews to sauces and gravies.

Very Veggie Soup

Ingredients:

- 4 tablespoons of olive oil (more if needed)
- 4 carrots, diced
- 4 celery stalks, diced
- 1 yellow onion, diced
- 6 cloves of garlic, minced
- 1 zucchini, chopped
- 1 squash, chopped
- 1 cup of baby spinach, chopped
- 1 jar of Rao's Marinade
- 8 cups of chicken broth (vegetable broth is an option)
- 1 tablespoon of dried oregano
- 1 tablespoon of cumin
- 1 tablespoon cinnamon
- 1 tablespoon chili powder
- Salt and pepper to taste

Preparation:

1. In a stock pot, add olive oil, sauté until soft, carrots, celery, onion, and garlic.
2. Once softened, add zucchini, squash and spinach.
3. Add one jar of Rao's marinade
4. Add 8 cups of broth
5. Add all seasonings
6. Let simmer for 2 hours, add more stock if necessary

Pea and Avocado Soup

Ingredients:

- 2 cups green peas shelled fresh or thaw out frozen peas
- 1 avocado
- 1 1/2 cups coconut water
- 1 1/2 teaspoons sea salt
- 1 tablespoon fresh basil
- 1 teaspoon black pepper
- 1 lemon juiced

Garnish

- dash of paprika
- 1 tablespoon fresh basil
- drizzle of extra virgin olive oil

Preparation:

1. Add all the ingredients into the blender and process until creamy.

2. Garnish with fresh basil, paprika and olive oil and serve.

Gazpacho Soup

Ingredients

- 3 large tomatoes
- 1 red pepper
- handful parsley
- 1/2 avocado
- 2 garlic cloves
- 1 cucumber
- 1/2 onion
- 2 tablespoons apple cider vinegar
- 1 teaspoon paprika
- 1 teaspoon sea salt
- 1/4 cup extra virgin olive oil

Garnish

- 1/2 avocado chopped
- 1/4 cup fresh cilantro

Preparation:

1. Add all the ingredients into the blender and process until creamy.
2. Refrigerate for 30 minutes then serve.

Butternut Squash Soup

Ingredients

- 2 cups water
- 2-3 cups raw butternut pumpkin
- 1 carrot
- 1 stem shallot
- 1/2 stem celery (with leaves)
- 1 small squash
- small knob ginger (with peel)
- 1 garlic clove (with peel)
- small piece chili
- handful cabbage
- 2-3 handful cashews
- 1 vegetarian stock cube
- small handful of herbs (parsley, rosemary, basil)

Preparation:

1. Put all the ingredients into the Vitamix container in the order listed and secure the lid.
2. Select speed 1, turn the machine on and quickly increase to the highest speed.
3. Use tamper to effectively press the ingredients into the blades if required whilst processing.
4. Blend for 5-6 minutes or until desired temperature is reached.
5. Stop the machine and serve.

Cucumber Avocado Gazpacho

Ingredients:

- 2 cucumbers, peeled and chopped
- 2 ripe avocados, peeled and chopped
- 1 green bell pepper, chopped
- 1 small red onion, chopped
- 2 cloves garlic, minced
- 2 cups vegetable broth
- 1/4 cup lime juice
- Salt and pepper, to taste
- Fresh cilantro leaves, for garnish

Preparation:

1. In a blender, combine cucumbers, avocados, green bell pepper, red onion, garlic, vegetable broth, and lime juice.
2. Blend until smooth.
3. Season with salt and pepper to taste.
4. Chill in the refrigerator for at least 1 hour.
5. Serve garnished with fresh cilantro leaves.

Chicken and Vegetable Soup

Ingredients:

- 1 lb boneless, skinless chicken breasts, diced into bite-sized pieces
- 2 tbsp olive oil

- 1 onion, diced
- 3 cloves garlic, minced
- 3 carrots, peeled and diced
- 2 stalks celery, diced
- 1 zucchini, diced
- 1 yellow squash, diced
- 1 red bell pepper, diced
- 1 can diced tomatoes, drained
- 4 cups low-sodium chicken broth
- 1 tsp dried thyme
- 1 tsp dried oregano
- Salt and pepper, to taste

Preparation:

1. In a large pot, heat the olive oil over medium-high heat. Add the chicken and cook until browned on all sides, about 5-7 minutes. Remove the chicken from the pot and set aside.
2. Add the onion and garlic to the pot and cook until softened, about 3-5 minutes.
3. Add the carrots, celery, zucchini, yellow squash, and red bell pepper to the pot and cook for 5-7 minutes, stirring occasionally, until the vegetables start to soften.
4. Add the diced tomatoes, chicken broth, thyme, oregano, and salt and pepper to the pot. Bring the soup to a boil, then reduce the heat to low and let it simmer for 20-25 minutes, or until the vegetables are tender.

5. Add the cooked chicken back into the pot and let it heat through for 2-3 minutes.
6. Serve the soup hot, garnished with fresh herbs or shredded Parmesan cheese, if desired.

Cucumber Watermelon Gazpacho

Ingredients:

- 4 cups watermelon, cubed and seeded
- 2 cups cucumber, peeled and chopped
- 1 small red bell pepper, chopped
- 1/2 small red onion, chopped
- 1/4 cup fresh basil leaves, chopped
- 3 tbsp fresh lime juice
- 1 tbsp white wine vinegar
- Salt and pepper, to taste
- 1/4 cup feta cheese, crumbled (optional)

Preparation:

1. In a blender, combine watermelon, cucumber, red bell pepper, red onion, basil, lime juice, and white wine vinegar. Blend until smooth.
2. Season with salt and pepper to taste.
3. Chill the soup for at least 1 hour before serving.
4. Garnish with feta cheese, if desired.

Chicken Soup

Ingredients:

- 1 tablespoon avocado oil or olive oil
- 6 cloves of garlic, minced
- 1 yellow onion, diced
- 2 large carrots, thinly sliced
- 2 celery stalks, roughly chopped
- 1 tablespoon fresh grated ginger
- 1 tablespoon fresh grated turmeric (or 1 teaspoon ground turmeric)
- 6 cups low sodium chicken broth
- 1 pound boneless skinless chicken breast or thighs
- 1 teaspoon freshly chopped rosemary
- 1 teaspoon freshly chopped thyme, stems removed
- ½ teaspoon salt
- Freshly ground black pepper
- 1 cup pearl or Israeli couscous
- 2/3 cup frozen peas (optional, but recommended)

Preparation:

1. Place a large dutch oven or pot over medium high heat and add in oil. Once oil is hot, add in garlic, onion, carrots and celery; cook for a few minutes until onion becomes translucent.
2. Next add in grated ginger and grated turmeric. Saute for 30 seconds to let the spices cook a bit, then add in

chicken broth, chicken breast, rosemary, thyme, salt and pepper.

3. Bring soup to a boil, then stir in couscous. You'll want the chicken to be covered by the broth so make sure you stir them down to the bottom.
4. Reduce heat to medium low and simmer uncovered for 20-25 minutes or until chicken is fully cooked.
5. Once chicken is cooked, remove with a slotted spoon and transfer to a cutting board to shred with two forks. Add chicken back to pot then stir in frozen peas. If you find that you don't have enough broth, feel free to add in another cup. Everyone likes their soup

Cucumber Gazpacho

Ingredients:

- 4 cups chopped cucumber
- 1 small onion, chopped
- 2 cloves garlic, minced
- 2 cups vegetable broth
- 1 cup Greek yogurt
- 1/4 cup fresh dill, chopped
- Salt and pepper, to taste

Preparation:

1. In a blender, combine cucumber, onion, garlic, and vegetable broth. Blend until smooth.
2. Stir in Greek yogurt and dill.

3. Season with salt and pepper.
4. Chill for at least 2 hours before serving.

Main Course

Broccoli and Garlic Stir Fry

Ingredients:

- 1/4 cup olive oil
- 6 cloves garlic, minced
- 1 bunch Broccoli florets (~4 cups; florets cut in half)
- 1/4 cup water

Preparation:

1. Heat the olive oil in a large sauté pan or skillet over medium heat. Add the minced garlic and saute until fragrant, about 30 seconds.
2. Add the broccoli florets. Season with salt and black pepper. Increase heat to medium high. Stir fry for about 3 minutes until the broccoli starts to turn bright green and brown a bit.
3. Add the water. Cover with a lid and cook for 2 minutes until broccoli is crisp-tender. (There will be steam under the lid.) Remove the lid and if there is any water remaining, stir fry for another minute until it evaporates. Adjust salt and pepper to taste if needed.

Lightly Sautéed Asparagus

Ingredients:

- 1 bunch of asparagus (about 1 1/4 lb.)
- 1 tbsp. olive oil
- 1 tbsp. unsalted butter

- 2 cloves garlic, chopped
- 1 lemon juice
- 2 tbsp. grated parmesan cheese, for serving

Preparation:

1. Trim the woody ends from the base of the asparagus spears by cutting off the bottom 2 inches or by snapping it off with your hands.
2. Blanch asparagus in boiling water for 3 to 4 minutes, then quickly transfer it to an ice bath. This is how to blanch asparagus properly so that it is crisp-tender and perfectly green.
3. Heat a large skillet over medium-high heat. Add the oil and swirl to coat the pan. Add the asparagus in a single layer and cook, turning occasionally, until lightly golden and almost tender, 8 to 10 minutes. (Cut a small piece from the end of one asparagus to see if it's near tender.)
4. Reduce the heat to low. Add the butter, garlic, salt and pepper and stir to coat the asparagus. Cook until the garlic is softened and fragrant, 1 to 2 more minutes. Immediately transfer to a serving plate.
5. Just before serving, squeeze the juice from the lemon half over the

Grilled Portabella Mushroom

Ingredients:

- 4 large portobello mushrooms *stems and gills removed, wiped clean*
- 1/4 cup balsamic vinegar
- 1 tablespoon olive oil
- 1 tablespoon low sodium soy sauce
- 1 tablespoon chopped fresh rosemary *or 1/2 teaspoon dried*
- 1 teaspoon garlic powder
- 1/2 teaspoon black pepper
- 1/8 teaspoon cayenne pepper *optional, plus additional to taste*
- Canola or vegetable oil *for grilling*

Preparation:

1. In a shallow baking dish, whisk together the balsamic vinegar, olive oil, soy sauce, rosemary, garlic powder, black pepper, and cayenne. Taste and adjust seasonings if you like. Add the mushrooms and turn to coat. Let sit for 5 minutes on one side, then flip and let sit 5 additional minutes. While the mushrooms marinate, prep the grill and anything you'd like to serve with them. You can let them sit for up to 30 minutes, so feel free to take your time—the longer they sit, the more intense the flavor will be.

2. Heat a grill or a large skillet over medium heat (about 350 to 400 degrees F). Brush the grill with oil to prevent sticking. Remove the mushrooms from the bowl, shaking off any excess marinade and reserving the marinade for basting. Cook on each side for 3-4 minutes, or until caramelized and deep golden brown. Brush the remaining marinade over the mushrooms several times as they cook.
3. Serve anyway you like. Options toast a hamburger bun.

Stuffed Portabella Mushroom

Ingredients:

- 4 portobello mushroom caps
- olive oil cooking spray
- 1 teaspoon Diamond Crystal kosher salt divided
- ¼ teaspoon black pepper divided
- 10 oz frozen chopped spinach
- 2 tablespoons olive oil
- 1 small onion finely chopped (6oz)
- 1 tablespoon minced fresh garlic
- ¼ cup dry-grated Parmesan

Preparation:

1. Preheat the broiler, setting the temperature to high (500 degrees F). Set an oven rack in the middle of the oven. Line a broiler-safe rimmed baking sheet with foil.

2. Gently wipe the mushrooms clean with a damp paper towel. Twist off or cut off the stem of each mushroom. Use a small spoon to scrape out the gills and discard them.
3. Spray the mushroom caps with olive oil on both sides. Sprinkle them with ½ teaspoon kosher salt and ⅛ teaspoon black pepper. Broil until just tender,
4. about 4 minutes per side. Place them upside down on paper towels to drain off any liquids.
5. Meanwhile, defrost the spinach in the microwave according to the directions on the package. Place the defrosted spinach in a colander to drain. Repeatedly press on the spinach with the back of a large spoon to remove as much water as possible.
6. Heat the olive oil in a large skillet over medium heat. Add the onion and cook it for 5-7 minutes, stirring occasionally, until golden. Add the garlic, spinach, ½ teaspoon kosher salt and ⅛ teaspoon black pepper and cook, stirring to combine everything, for 1-2 more minutes. Remove the skillet from the heat and allow it to cool for a couple of minutes, then mix in the Parmesan.
7. Evenly distribute the spinach mixture among the mushrooms. Don't press down on the filling - it's prettier when it's piled high on top of the mushrooms.

8. Place the stuffed mushrooms back under the broiler (on the middle rack) for 2-3 minutes, until the filling is golden. Serve immediately.

Okra and Olive Oil

The entire okra plant is edible. The leaves can be eaten raw in salads or cooked like any other greens. Okra pods can even be eaten raw. The less cooked okra is, the better it is for you.

Ingredients

- 1 pound fresh okra, no need to slice, leave whole
- Drizzle of olive oil

Vegan Chili

Ingredients

- 3 cups tomatoes, diced (I used grape)
- 1 small red bell pepper (orange would be great too), diced
- 1 large rib of celery, diced
- 1/2 red onion, diced
- 1 small zucchini, diced
- 1 corn off the cob
- 1 – 2 cloves garlic, minced
- chopped cilantro, chopped (use as much as you like)
- 2 teaspoons chili powder, to taste
- 1 teaspoon cumin

- 1 teaspoon oregano, fresh or dried
- 1/4 teaspoon sea salt, to taste

Vegan Meat

- 1 cup walnuts
- cup mushrooms
- 1 tablespoon cumin
- 2 teaspoons coriander
- 1 teaspoon tamari, coconut amino's, bragg's or 1/4 teaspoon sea salt, to taste

Preparation:

1. Vegetables: Prepare vegetables and combine all ingredients in large size bowl. Place 1/2 or so of the mix into a food processor and blend until pureed. Return puree to diced vegetables and toss well.
2. Nut Meat: Place all ingredients into food processor and pulse until crumbly. You don't want to over blend or it will be a paste.
3. Serve: Place vegetable chili in bowls and top with nut meat adding any additional garnishes you like.

Zucchini Noodles with Pesto

Ingredients:

- 4 medium zucchinis, spiralized
- 1 cup fresh basil leaves
- 1/4 cup pine nuts

- 1/4 cup grated Parmesan cheese
- 2 cloves garlic
- 1/3 cup olive oil
- Salt and pepper, to taste

Preparation:

1. In a food processor, combine basil, pine nuts, Parmesan, garlic, salt, and pepper. Process until smooth.
2. With the processor running, slowly drizzle in olive oil to create a smooth pesto.
3. Toss zucchini noodles with pesto and serve immediately.

Zucchini Noodle Caprese

Ingredients:

- 4 medium zucchini, spiralized
- 2 cups cherry tomatoes, halved
- 1 cup fresh mozzarella pearls
- 1/2 cup fresh basil leaves, chopped
- 1/4 cup extra-virgin olive oil
- 3 tbsp balsamic vinegar
- Salt and pepper, to taste

Preparation:

1. In a large bowl, combine zucchini noodles, cherry tomatoes, mozzarella pearls, and basil.

2. In a small bowl, whisk together olive oil and balsamic vinegar. Season with salt and pepper.
3. Pour the dressing over the zucchini noodle mixture and toss to combine.

Cauliflower Fried "Rice" with Pineapple

Ingredients:

- 1 large head cauliflower, riced
- 1 tbsp coconut oil
- 1 small onion, chopped
- 2 cloves garlic, minced
- 1/2 cup frozen peas
- 1/2 cup diced carrots
- 1/2 cup diced pineapple
- 2 eggs, beaten
- 3 tbsp low-sodium soy sauce
- 2 green onions, sliced
- 1/4 cup chopped cilantro

Instructions:

1. In a large skillet or wok, heat coconut oil over medium heat.

Grilled Pineapple Skewers

Ingredients:

- 1 pineapple, peeled and cut into chunks
- 2 tablespoons honey
- 1 tablespoon lime juice
- 1/2 teaspoon ground cinnamon
- Pinch of salt
- Wooden skewers, soaked in water for 30 minutes

Preparation:

1. Preheat grill to medium heat.
2. In a small bowl, whisk together honey, lime juice, cinnamon, and salt.
3. Thread pineapple chunks onto skewers.
4. Brush pineapple skewers with honey mixture.
5. Grill for 5-7 minutes, turning occasionally, until pineapple is caramelized.
6. Serve hot.

SMOOTHIES

Berry Blast Smoothie

- 1 cup mixed frozen berries
- 1/2 banana
- 1 cup unsweetened almond milk
- 1 tablespoon chia seeds
- 1/2 teaspoon honey (optional)
- Blend all ingredients until smooth and enjoy!

Green Machine Smoothie

- 1 cup spinach
- 1/2 cup kale
- 1/2 avocado
- 1/2 banana
- 1 cup unsweetened almond milk
- 1 tablespoon honey (optional)
- Juice of 1/2 lemon
- Blend all ingredients until smooth and enjoy!

Tropical Paradise Smoothie

- 1/2 cup frozen pineapple
- 1/2 cup frozen mango
- 1/2 banana
- 1 cup unsweetened coconut milk
- 1 tablespoon unsweetened shredded coconut

- Juice of 1/2 lime
- Blend all ingredients until smooth and enjoy!

Chocolate Peanut Butter Smoothie:

- 1 banana
- 1 tablespoon peanut butter
- 1 tablespoon cocoa powder
- 1 cup unsweetened almond milk
- 1/2 teaspoon vanilla extract
- 1/2 teaspoon honey (optional)
- Blend all ingredients until smooth and enjoy!

Vanilla Berry Protein Smoothie

- 1 scoop vanilla protein powder
- 1/2 cup mixed frozen berries
- 1/2 banana
- 1 cup unsweetened almond milk
- 1 tablespoon chia seeds
- Blend all ingredients until smooth and enjoy!

Popeye Smoothie

- 1 cup spinach
- 1 ripe banana
- 1 scoop vanilla protein powder

- 1 tablespoon chia seeds
- 1 cup unsweetened almond milk
- Ice cubes (optional)

Blend all the ingredients together until smooth and enjoy!

Blueberry and Kale Smoothie

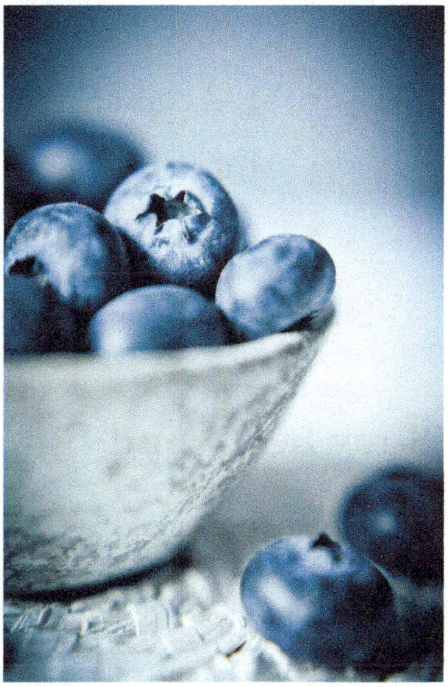

- 1 cup fresh kale
- 1/2 cup frozen blueberries
- 1/2 banana
- 1 tablespoon almond butter
- 1/2 cup plain Greek yogurt
- 1/2 cup unsweetened almond milk

Blend all the ingredients until smooth and creamy.

Mango and Pineapple Smoothie

- 1 cup frozen mango chunks
- 1/2 cup frozen pineapple chunks
- 1/2 banana
- 1/2 cup coconut milk

- 1/2 cup orange juice

Blend all the ingredients until smooth and serve chilled.

Banana and Oatmeal Smoothie

- 1 ripe banana
- 1/2 cup rolled oats
- 1/2 cup plain Greek yogurt
- 1/2 cup unsweetened almond milk
- 1 teaspoon honey
- A pinch of cinnamon

Blend all the ingredients together until smooth and enjoy.

Strawberry and Banana Smoothie

- 1 ripe banana
- 1/2 cup frozen strawberries
- 1/2 cup plain Greek yogurt
- 1/2 cup unsweetened almond milk
- 1 teaspoon honey

Blend all the ingredients together until smooth and serve immediately.

Green Detox Smoothie

- 1 cup spinach
- 1/2 cucumber
- 1/2 avocado
- 1/2 green apple
- 1/2 lemon, juiced
- 1/2 cup coconut water
- 1/2 cup ice cubes

Blend all the ingredients until smooth.

Berry Berry Good Smoothie

- 1 cup mixed berries (strawberries, raspberries, blueberries)
- 1 banana
- 1/2 cup plain Greek yogurt
- 1/2 cup almond milk
- 1/2 teaspoon honey (optional)
- 1/2 cup ice cubes

Blend all the ingredients until smooth.

Cabo Smoothie

- 1 cup chopped pineapple
- 1 banana
- 1/2 cup chopped mango

- 1/2 cup coconut water
- 1/2 cup plain Greek yogurt
- 1/2 cup ice cubes

Blend all the ingredients until smooth.

Chocolate Banana Smoothie

- 1 banana
- 1 tablespoon cocoa powder
- 1 tablespoon almond butter
- 1/2 cup almond milk
- 1/2 teaspoon vanilla extract
- 1/2 cup ice cubes

Blend all the ingredients until smooth.

Peanut Butter and Jelly Smoothie

- 1 cup frozen mixed berries
- 1 banana
- 1/4 cup peanut butter
- 1/2 cup almond milk
- 1/2 teaspoon honey (optional)
- 1/2 cup ice cubes

Blend all the ingredients until smooth.

Celery Smoothie

Ingredients

- 4 medium ribs celery (¾ cup chopped)
- 1 large green apple
- 1 banana
- ½ teaspoon peeled and grated ginger (from fresh ginger root)
- 2 cups baby spinach leaves
- ½ cup water
- 10 ice cubes
- 1 ½ tablespoons fresh squeezed lemon juice (1/2 lemon)

Preparation:

1. Roughly chop the celery. Chop the apple into chunks, leaving the peel on. Break the banana into pieces. Peel and grate or mince the ginger.
2. Place everything in a blender and blend until smooth, stopping and scraping as necessary and adding a splash more water if it's too thick. Drink immediately or store for up to 1 day.

Strawberry, Blueberry Smoothie

Ingredients:

- cup frozen strawberries
- 1 cup frozen blueberries
- 1 banana (room temperature)
- ¼ cup Greek yogurt*
- 1 cup milk (or almond milk or oat milk)
- 1 tablespoon maple syrup, honey, or agave syrup
- ½ cup ice
- 1/4 to 1/2 teaspoon cinnamon*

Preparation:

1. Place all ingredients in a blender, breaking the banana into pieces. Blend until creamy and frothy, stopping and scraping down the sides as necessary. If desired, garnish with a strawberry and blueberries.

JUICES

Green Juice

- 2 green apples
- 1 cucumber
- 1/2 lemon (peeled)
- 1 inch ginger
- 2 cups kale

Beetroot Juice

- 2 beetroots
- 1 carrot
- 1 orange (peeled)
- 1 inch ginger

Carrot Juice

- 4-5 carrots
- 1/2 lemon (peeled)
- 1 inch ginger
- 1 apple

Pineapple and Turmeric Juice

- 1/4 pineapple
- 1/2 inch turmeric root
- 1/2 lemon (peeled)
- 1/4 tsp black pepper

Citrus Juice

- 2 oranges (peeled)
- 1/2 grapefruit (peeled)
- 1 lemon (peeled)
- 1 inch ginger

Celery Juice

Ingredients:

- 8 medium-large stalks of celery (about 1 bunch)
- 1 large green apple
- ½ cup water
- 1 teaspoon lemon or lime juice (optional)

Preparation:

1. Roughly chop the celery. Chop the apple, keeping the skin on.
2. Place the celery, apple, and water in a blender. Blend on high until pureed and a juice forms.
3. Pass the juice through a fine mesh sieve or a nut milk bag to strain out the pulp. Discard the pulp (or use: see ideas above). Stir in the fresh lemon juice (add more if desired). Drink immediately over ice, or chill before drinking.

Green Earth Juice

- 2 cups spinach
- 1 green apple
- 1 cucumber
- 1 lemon (juiced)
- 1 inch piece of ginger (peeled) Blend all the ingredients together in a juicer or blender until smooth. This juice is rich in vitamins A and C, and antioxidants.

Carrot-Orange Juice

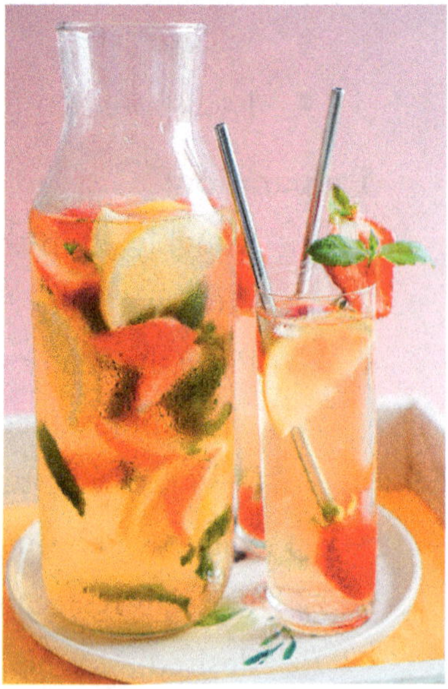

- 4 medium-sized carrots
- 2 oranges
- 1 inch piece of ginger (peeled) Juice the carrots and oranges together and then add ginger to taste. This juice is loaded with vitamin C and beta-carotene, which is great for your skin and immune system.

Beetroot-Apple Juice

- 1 medium-sized beetroot
- 2 green apples
- 1 inch piece of ginger (peeled)
- 1 lemon (juiced) Juice the beetroot and apples together, and then add ginger and lemon juice. This juice is rich in antioxidants, iron, and vitamin C.

Pineapple-Cucumber Juice

- 1 cup pineapple chunks
- 1 medium-sized cucumber
- 1 lime (juiced)
- 1 handful of mint leaves Juice the pineapple and cucumber together, then add lime juice and blend with mint leaves. This juice is a great source of vitamin C and helps with digestion.

Watermelon-Lime Juice

- 2 cups watermelon (seedless)
- 1 lime (juiced)
- 1 handful of mint leaves Blend the watermelon in a blender, then add lime juice and mint leaves. This juice is high in antioxidants, vitamin C, and is also hydrating.
-

Beet-Berry Blast

- 1 small beet
- 1 cup mixed berries (strawberries, raspberries, blueberries)
- 1 small orange, peeled

Preparation:

Wash and prep all ingredients. Run them through a juicer and enjoy!

Pineapple-Cucumber Cooler

- 1/4 fresh pineapple, peeled
- 1 small cucumber
- 1/2 lime, peeled
- 1 small handful of mint leaves

Preparation:

Wash and prep all ingredients. Run them through a juicer and enjoy!

Watermelon-Mint Refresher

- 1/4 small seedless watermelon
- 1 small handful of mint leaves
- 1/2 lime, peeled

Preparation:

Wash and prep all ingredients. Run them through a juicer and enjoy!

Grilled Peach with Greek Yogurt and Honey

Ingredients:

- 2 ripe peaches
- 1 cup Greek yogurt
- 2 tbsp honey
- Cinnamon (optional)

Preparation:

1. Preheat a grill or grill pan over medium heat.
2. Cut peaches in half and remove the pit.
3. Grill the peaches for 3-4 minutes on each side, or until grill marks appear.
4. In a small bowl, mix the Greek yogurt and honey together.
5. Serve the grilled peaches with a dollop of the yogurt mixture on top.
6. Sprinkle with cinnamon, if desired.

Watermelon Sorbet

Ingredients:

- 6 cups cubed seedless watermelon
- 6 tablespoons sugar

- 3 tablespoons lime juice
- 1 cup ice

Preparation:

Chop the watermelon into cubes.

1. Place in a blender and blend until a smooth juice forms, then add ice and blend again.
2. Pour the mixture into an ice cream maker and freeze for 20 to 25 minutes. The texture will be icy and creamy at this point. If desired, place in a container and freeze for 1 hour for a harder texture that forms into scoops. You can freeze up to 2 hours day of (stir before serving). Freezing overnight makes a very icy texture. If you have leftovers the next day, allow them to sit at room temperature for about 20 minutes. To improve the texture, you can pulse in a blender or food processor if desired.

Berry and Yogurt Parfait

Ingredients:

- 1 cup plain Greek yogurt
- 1 cup mixed berries (strawberries, blueberries, raspberries)
- 2 tbsp granola

Preparation:

1. In a glass or jar, layer the Greek yogurt and mixed berries.

2. Repeat until the glass or jar is full.
3. Top with granola.

Vegan Strawberry Ice Cream

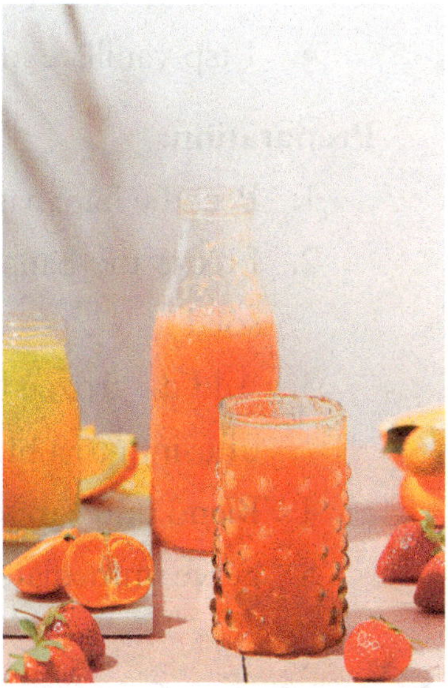

Ingredients

- Cream from the tops of 2 13.66-ounce cans of full-fat coconut milk
- 3 cups frozen chopped strawberries
- 1/3 cup maple syrup
- 1/4 teaspoon vanilla extract

Preparation:

1. To make vegan ice cream, you need: 2 (13- to 15-ounce) cans full-fat coconut milk; 1/2 cup agave, honey, turbinado sugar, or cane sugar; 1/4 teaspoon salt; 2 tablespoons cornstarch (or 1 tablespoon arrowroot starch); 1 1/2 teaspoons vanilla extract
2. At least 24 hours before you plan to churn the ice cream, put the ice cream machine's bowl in the freezer to freeze. It should be frozen solid before using (you should hear no liquid sloshing inside when you shake it).

Banana Nice Cream

Ingredients:

- 2 ripe bananas
- 1/4 cup milk (any kind)
- 1 tsp vanilla extract (optional)

Preparation:

1. Peel the bananas and cut them into chunks.
2. Freeze the banana chunks for at least 2 hours or until solid.
3. Add the frozen banana chunks, milk, and vanilla extract (if using) to a blender or food processor.
4. Blend until smooth and creamy.
5. Serve immediately or freeze for later.

Mango and Coconut Chia Pudding

Ingredients

- 1/4 cup chia seeds
- 1 cup coconut milk
- 1 ripe mango, peeled and diced
- 1 tbsp honey (optional)

Preparation:

1. In a bowl, whisk together the chia seeds and coconut milk.
2. Cover and refrigerate for at least 2 hours or overnight.

3. In a blender or food processor, blend the diced mango until smooth.
4. Stir the honey into the chia pudding.
5. Layer the chia pudding and mango puree in a glass or jar.
6. Chill until ready to serve.

Baked Apples with Cinnamon and Walnuts

Ingredients:

- 2 apples, cored and sliced
- 1 tsp cinnamon
- 1/4 cup chopped walnuts
- 2 tbsp maple syrup

Preparation:

1. Preheat the oven to 375°F.
2. In a bowl, mix the sliced apples, cinnamon, and chopped walnuts together.
3. Transfer the mixture to a baking dish.
4. Drizzle the maple syrup over the top.
5. Bake for 20-25 minutes or until the apples are tender.
6. Serve warm.

100 Water-Enhancing Recipes

Drinking plain water can sometimes feel monotonous. This chapter is dedicated to providing you with simple, delicious recipes that add flavor and excitement to your water while still keeping you hydrated.

Here's a fun fact: 25% of Americans don't like the taste of water. So if you're one of them, it may be time to try something new. A healthy and nutritious way to drink your H2O, infusing your water with fruit, vegetables or herbs will add flavor and nutrients (without resorting to chemicals or artificial sweeteners).

Choose your fruits, herbs, and vegetables. You can use any combination of ingredients you like, but some popular options include:

- Citrus fruits such as lemons, limes, and oranges
- Berries such as strawberries, blueberries, and raspberries
- Cucumber
- Mint, basil, or rosemary
- Ginger
- Watermelon
- Pineapple
- Apples

Basic instruction for flavor infusion:

The key to taste great water is by infusing it with fruit and herbs. I love fresh fruit, but frozen fruits are good too if the produce is out of season. Wash your fruit before use in order to remove any harmful substances that may have contaminated it during the harvest or storage process.

To wash your fruit:

use a spray bottle filled with 3 cups of water and 1 cup of white vinegar, spray each piece of fruit with about six quarts of the solution, just enough to coat the service, and then rinse it under tap water and dry it with a clean paper towel. Wash the produce before peeling it so dirt and bacteria aren't transferring from the knife to the fruit or vegetable.

Slice your ingredients into thin slices or small pieces. You can leave the skins on or remove them as desired.

Add your sliced ingredients to the pitcher or jar. Use a spoon or muddler to gently mash them a bit to release their flavors. Add 1 to 2 cups of fruit; you can double the recipe by using a 2 quart or more container, depending on how much flavor you want for the glass.

Fill the pitcher or jar with water. Use filtered or tap water that has been left to sit out for a few hours to allow any chlorine to evaporate.

Cover the pitcher or jar with a lid and refrigerate for at least 2-4 hours, or overnight, to allow the flavors to infuse into the water.

When you're ready to serve, give the water a stir and pour it over ice, if desired. You can strain the water through a strainer or cheesecloth to remove any solids before serving.

Many people ask if they can reuse the pulp that is left behind? The answer is to taste it, it typically doesn't have much flavor. Depending on the fruit or vegetable I use, I will add it to my dogs food. Or add it to your compost pile.

Enjoy your refreshing infused water! You can keep it in the fridge for up to 2-3 days.

Tips:

- Experiment with different ingredient combinations to find your favorite flavors.
- Use organic fruits and vegetables whenever possible to avoid pesticides and other harmful chemicals.

- If you want a stronger flavor, let the water infuse for longer or use more ingredients.
- You can also add a touch of honey or agave syrup to sweeten the water if desired.

And don't worry about getting bored—there are literally hundreds of combinations to keep things interesting!

Herbs

can add a layer of depth to your water. Of course, it's up to you and your taste buds, but many herbs complement fruit flavors. The same rule applies to herbs; buy organic and wash your herbs thoroughly.

1. Mint

Mint is a good digestive aid. Just boiling a few leaves in water, straining them and drinking the water after it cools down, can help your food get digested better. The less detox work your skin has to do, the better it will look.

2. Basil

Basil has anti-inflammatory properties that can prevent inflammation, making your skin look younger. The flavonoids present in basil also protect the skin from damage. Drink water infused with basil leaves for best results.

3. Lemon

Squeeze lemon juice on your bowl of fruit, or your salad and as a finishing touch to your curries. Lemon juice has vitamin C, which is known to boost collagen and clean the liver. Clean liver results in cleaner and brighter looking skin.

4. Ginger

Ginger, as we all know, has multiple benefits. Adding ginger to your tea, boiling it and drinking the concoction, or adding to your food, can help with digestion and inflammation.

5. Cinnamon

If you are diabetic or have a tendency to binge on the sweet stuff, drinking water infused with cinnamon sticks left overnight, can help stabilize fluctuating blood sugar levels, improve blood circulation and prevent pimples and zits.

6. Juice Cubes

Sugar is known to cause premature aging. If you like to drink pre-packaged juices, but want to cut down on the sugar, freeze a few cubes of your favorite fruit juice (homemade) in an ice tray. Pour into your bottle of water so you get the fruity flavors without the excess sugar.

7. Raw Honey And Apple Cider Vinegar

Adding a few drops of raw honey or a tablespoon of organic Apple Cider Vinegar to your glass of water can help clear acne from your skin and prevent further breakouts.

Sweetened or spice up your water.

- Stevia leaves are a great way to naturally add sweetness to your water; if you're using the liquid or powder Stevia, remember that two tablespoons of Stevia equal 1 cup of sugar. Add honey agave nectar Stevia or Monk fruit if you're using the hot method. Other natural sweeteners are:
- Maple syrup
- Honey
- Agave nectar
- Coconut sugar

DIY Water

Making your own vitamin water is a delicious and hydrating way to get some extra nutrients into your day. This recipe focuses on natural ingredients rich in vitamins and antioxidants, providing a refreshing and healthy alternative to store-bought drinks. Here's how to make it:

Ingredients:

- 6 cups of filtered water
- 2 cups of mixed fresh fruit (e.g., berries, citrus slices, kiwi, and mango)
- Fresh herbs (e.g., mint, basil, or rosemary for added flavor)

- 1-2 tablespoons of honey or agave syrup (optional, for sweetness)

Instructions:

1. **Prepare the Fruit:** Wash the fruit thoroughly. Slice any larger fruits into thin slices or wedges. Berries can be left whole. The variety of fruits used can be tailored to your preference or nutritional goals. For example, citrus fruits are high in vitamin C, while berries offer antioxidants.
2. **Mix Water and Fruit:** In a large pitcher, combine the filtered water with the prepared fruit. Use a spoon to gently press the fruit against the side of the pitcher to release some of the juices for extra flavor.
3. **Add Herbs:** Add a handful of fresh herbs to the pitcher. Mint is a popular choice for its refreshing taste, but basil or rosemary can add unique and delightful flavors. Lightly bruise the leaves with your fingers before adding them to help release their oils.
4. **Sweeten (Optional):** If you prefer a slightly sweeter drink, stir in honey or agave syrup to taste. This step is optional and can be adjusted based on personal preference.
5. **Chill:** Cover the pitcher and refrigerate for at least 2-4 hours, allowing the flavors to infuse. For best results, you can leave it to infuse overnight.

6. **Serve:** Stir the vitamin water well before serving. Pour over ice if desired, making sure to get some of the fruit and herbs into each glass for added appeal.
7. **Storage:** Keep the vitamin water refrigerated and consume within 2-3 days for best freshness and flavor.

Tips:

- **Experiment with Combinations:** Create your own blends based on what's in season or your nutritional needs. For instance, lemon and lime for detoxifying properties, or cucumber and mint for a cooling summer drink.
- **Enhance with Supplements:** For an extra vitamin boost, consider dissolving a vitamin C or B-complex tablet in the water. However, be mindful of daily recommended intakes to avoid excessive consumption.
- **Stay Hydrated:** Homemade vitamin water is a great way to stay hydrated while enjoying a burst of natural flavor and nutrients. It's a healthier alternative to sugary sodas and commercial drinks.

"Gatorade" Electrolyte Water

Making your own "Gatorade" at home is a simple and effective way to stay hydrated, especially during workouts or hot weather. This homemade sports drink recipe aims to replace electrolytes lost through sweat, using natural ingredients. Here's how you can make it:

Ingredients:

- 1/4 cup freshly squeezed lemon juice
- 1/4 cup freshly squeezed lime juice
- 2 cups water (still or sparkling for a fizzy alternative)
- 1/8 tsp salt (preferably Himalayan pink salt for its trace minerals)
- 2 tablespoons honey or maple syrup (adjust to taste for sweetness)

Optional Additions for Flavor and Electrolytes:

- 1/4 cup orange juice (for additional vitamins and flavor)
- A pinch of magnesium powder or calcium powder (for added electrolytes)

Instructions:

1. **Juice Preparation:** Begin by squeezing the lemons and limes until you have 1/4 cup of juice from each. If you're adding orange juice, prepare that as well.
2. **Mix the Ingredients:** In a pitcher, combine the freshly squeezed lemon and lime juices with the water. Stir in the salt and honey (or maple syrup). The salt replaces sodium lost through sweat, and the honey adds a natural sweetness while providing some energy.
3. **Dissolve the Sweetener:** Stir the mixture vigorously until the honey (or maple syrup) and salt are completely

dissolved. This step is crucial for a smooth drinking experience.

4. **Add Optional Ingredients:** If you're using orange juice or any optional powders (like magnesium or calcium), add them now and stir well to combine.
5. **Chill:** Refrigerate the mixture until it's cold. Serving it chilled enhances its refreshment factor, especially after a workout or on a hot day.
6. **Serve:** Serve the homemade "Gatorade" over ice if desired, or take it with you in a reusable water bottle for on-the-go hydration.

Coldwater recipes

For each one of these recipes prepare the fruit/vegetable as stated and muddle gently.

Add 16 ounces of water to each of the following recipes.

Refrigerate leftover infused water within 2 hours. Fresh infused water should be stored in a tightly covered container in the refrigerator for about two days. Prior to drinking, be sure to inspect the water for any spoilage.

Note:

Prepare your fruit prior to infusion to make sure your water is free of any contaminants that can cause food poisoning.

In a large pitcher, place the desired combination of fruit or herbs.

Add ice and fill container with water. Add additional fruit or herbs to garnish, if desired.

- Cucumber, citrus fruits, and fresh herbs work best for infusion. They hold up well over time and infuse flavor quickly. Citrus rinds can make a bitter flavor after 1 day, so you may want to remove the rinds.
- Infuse the water for 1 hour, and enjoy the best flavor within 1 day. Some waters like cucumber water can last for up to 3 days.
- The longer they rest, the stronger the flavor. Within about 15 minutes, you'll get a nice, mild flavor of whatever you're infusing the water with. The longer it infuses, the stronger the flavor will get.
- You can reuse the fruit for more batches. I can normally get about four refills before the flavor of the fruit is all gone. Keep refilling that pitcher or carafe! I like to make up a carafe in the morning, refill it throughout the day, and then compost the fruit before bed. The flavor will fade after each refill, but it'll still be delicious. Once your fruit has lost all its flavor, compost it.
- The nutritional benefit is increased hydration. Infusing water with fruit might add a negligible amount of vitamins and minerals from the fruit, but the real nutritional benefit is to make you want to drink more water! Hydration is good.
- Drink it that day. For the best flavor, drink it the day you make it—you might be able to get by with 36 hours,

depending on how fresh your fruit is, but it's best to make it when you want to drink it. For citrus fruits with peel, you want to drink it within a few hours or the water tends to get bitter.

- You can use sparkling or regular water. Use whatever kind of water makes you happy. Sparkling water makes everything feel a bit more fancy, doesn't it?

The following recipes are for a 16 ounce pitcher of water (double the ingredients if using a larger pitcher).

Apple and cinnamon: Slice an apple with a cinnamon stick.

Apricot and basil: Slice a ripe apricot and a few sprigs of fresh basil.

Black and blue water. Handful of blackberries and blueberries.

Blueberry water. One cup of blueberries and a touch of honey.

Blackberry and sage: Add a handful of fresh blackberries and a few sprigs of fresh sage.

Blackberry water. Handful of blackberries, Stevia (optional).

Blackberry, cucumber, and orange water. Handful of blackberries, a few slices of cucumber, and one orange quartered.

Blackberry, lemon water. Handful blackberries, one lemon sliced sweetened with a small amount of honey or Stevia or monk fruit.

Blackberry, lemon, and ginger water. Handful of blackberries, one lemon slice, and 1/8 inch of grated ginger.

Blackberry, orange, and rosemary water. Handful of blackberries, one orange sliced, one sprig of rosemary.

Blackberry, sage water. Handful of blackberries and one sage leaf.

Blueberry and basil: Add a handful of fresh blueberries and a few sprigs of basil.

Blueberry and lemon water. Handful of blueberries and one lemon quartered.

Blueberry fennel water. Handful of blueberries and ¼ cup chopped fennel.

Blueberry Ginger water. Handful of blueberries and quarter-inch fresh ginger grated.

Blueberry mint water. Handful of blueberries and six mint leaves.

Blueberry, watermelon, and peach water. Handful of blueberries, ¼ cup of watermelon, and 1 peach quartered.

Cantaloupe, berry, and ginger water. ¼ cup ripe cantaloupe, 1/4cup mixed berries, and 1/4 inch grated fresh ginger.

Cantaloupe, strawberry water. ¼ cup ripe cantaloupe and ¼ cup strawberries.

Cardamom, orange water. Four cardamom pods and one orange quartered.

Cherry water. One handful of dark cherries.

Cherry and lemon: Add sliced cherries and a sliced lemon.

Cherry, basil water. Handful of dark cherries and six basil leaves.

Cherry, lime water. Handful of dark cherries, one lime quartered, Stevia or monk fruit optional.

Coconut, pineapple water. One cup coconut water and ½ cup pineapple.

Cranberry and orange: Add fresh cranberries and a sliced orange.

Cranberry cinnamon water. One cup of frozen cranberries, and add half a cinnamon stick.

Cranberry water. One cup of frozen cranberries.

Cucumber and mint: Slice half a cucumber and add it to a pitcher of water with a handful of fresh mint leaves.

Cucumber apple and lemon water. One half of a cucumber, one apple sliced, one lemon slice.

Cucumber basil water. One cucumber slice, and eight basil leaves.

Cucumber honeydew and cantaloupe water. 1/2 cucumbers sliced, 1/2 cup honeydew, 1/2 cut up cantaloupe.

Cucumber lemon and ginger water. ½ cucumber sliced, one lemon sliced, and 1/4 inch grated ginger.

Cucumber lemon and mint water. ½ cucumber sliced, one lemon slice, and six mint leaves.

Cucumber lemon rosemary and mint water. ½ cucumber sliced, one lemon sliced, one sprig of rosemary and six mint leaves.

Cucumber rosemary and fennel water. One cucumber sliced, one sprig of rosemary and two fennel tops.

Cucumber water. ½ cucumber sliced.

Cucumber, strawberry water. ½ cucumber sliced and 1/2 cup strawberries.

Grapefruit and mint water. One grapefruit peeled and quartered, 4 mint leaves.

Grapefruit and rosemary. One grapefruit peeled and quartered, and a few sprigs of fresh rosemary.

Grapefruit apple fennel and mint water. One grapefruit peeled and quartered, 1 apple quartered ,one three-inch fennel stalk, six mint leaves.

Grapefruit pineapple, orange, and cinnamon water. One grapefruit peeled and quartered, juice from canned pineapple, one orange quartered, and one cinnamon stick.

Grapefruit water. One grapefruit, peeled and quartered.

Green apple citrus water. One green apple slice, one orange slice, and one lemon sliced.

Green apple water. One green apple sliced.

Honeydew melon and mint water. ½ cup ripe honeydew melon and six mint leaves.

Honeydew melon water. One cup ripe honeydew melon.

Kiwi and mint: Slice one kiwi and 4 fresh mint leaves.

Kiwi mint and mango water. One kiwi peeled, one mango peeled, and six mint leaves.

Kiwi rosemary water. One ripe kiwi peeled, one sprig of rosemary.

Lemon and chia Water. Squeeze one lemon, add one tablespoon of chia seeds to water.

Lemon and ginger: Slice one lemon and a few pieces of fresh ginger root.

Lemon basil water. 1 lemon sliced, eight basil leaves, Stevia or monk fruit optional.

Lemon cucumber water. 1 lemon sliced, ½ cucumber sliced.

Lemongrass, and mint water. One 2 in cut lemongrass, six mint leaves.

Lemon ginger water. 1 lemon sliced, 1/8 inch grated ginger.

Lemon mint water. 1 lemon sliced six mint leaves.

Lemon rosemary water. 1 lemon sliced, one sprig of rosemary.

Lemon thyme water. One lemon sliced, one sprig thyme.

Lemon water. 1 Lemon sliced.

Lime cilantro water. One lime slice, three sprigs of cilantro.

Lime mint water. 1 lime sliced, six mint leaves.

Lime orange and mint water. One lime sliced, one orange piece, and six mint leaves.

Lime water. 2 limes sliced.

Lychee pineapple water. One lychee with syrup and 1 cup pineapple.

Lychee water. One can of lychee with syrup, just add water.

Mango and ginger. One fresh mango cut into small pieces and 1/8 inch grated ginger.

Mango kiwi water. One cup mango, one kiwi, peeled.

Mango water. 1 cup chopped mango.

Mango, basil water. 1 cup mango, peeled and cubed, 6 basil leaves.

Mango, Raspberry, and Ginger. 1 mango peeled and cubed, 1/2 cup raspberries 1 (2-inch) piece fresh ginger peeled and thinly sliced.

Mint water. Six mint leaves. Try a variety of mint leaves, like spearmint, peppermint, or chocolate mint.

Orange and cinnamon: Slice one orange and add one cinnamon stick.

Orange basil water. One orange sliced, six basil leaves.

Orange Water. Slice 1 orange with juice.

Orange, blueberry and lemon water. One orange slice, 1/4 cup blueberries, one lemon sliced.

Passion fruit water. Slice one passion fruit.

Peach and thyme: Slice one ripe peach with a few sprigs of fresh thyme.

Peach melon and rosemary water. One cup of peaches, 1 cup of any type of melon, and one sprig of rosemary.

Peach raspberry water. One half-cup peaches and ¼ cup raspberries.

Pear and thyme: Slice one ripe pear one sprig of fresh thyme.

Pineapple and rosemary: ½ cup fresh or canned pineapple with a few sprigs of fresh rosemary.

Pineapple and coconut water. One cup of canned pineapple, one cup coconut water.

Pineapple cilantro water. One cup pineapple, fresh or canned, one sprig of cilantro.

Pineapple lime water. One cup of canned pineapple + juice, one lime slice.

Pineapple mango sage and blackberry water. One half-cup pineapple, 1/2 cup mango sliced, for sage leaves, 1/2 cup blueberries.

Pineapple mint water. One cup of canned pineapple plus juice, six mint leaves.

Pineapple water. One cup of pineapple from the can with juice.

Plum and sage: Slice a ripe plum with a few sprigs of fresh sage.

Pomegranate and mint: Add pomegranate seeds and a handful of fresh mint leaves.

Pomegranate Blueberry water. One cup pomegranate juice plus seeds, ½ cup blueberries.

Pomegranate orange water. One cup of pomegranate, one slice of orange.

Raspberry and lime: Add a handful of fresh raspberries and one sliced lime .t

Raspberry fennel water. ½ cup of raspberries, one fennel top.

Raspberry green apple water. ½ cup raspberries, one green apple slice.

Raspberry lime water. ½ cup raspberries, 1 lime slice.

Raspberry rose and vanilla water. ½ cup raspberries, six organic rose petals or rose water, ¼ vanilla bean.

Rosewater. Middle Eastern stores carry organic rose petals or purchase a bottle of rosewater and add ten drops of rosewater to 1 quart of water.

Strawberry and thyme: 6 sliced strawberries and a few sprigs of fresh thyme.

Strawberry basil water. ½ cup strawberries, and six basil leaves.

Strawberry kiwi. ½ cup strawberry, one peeled kiwi, sliced.

Strawberry lemon water. ½ cup of strawberries, one lemon sliced.

Strawberry lime water. ½ cup of strawberries, and one lime slice.

Strawberry orange water. ½ cup strawberries, one orange slice.

Strawberry peach mint water. 1/2 cup strawberries, 1/2 cup peaches, and six mint leaves.

Strawberry pomegranate and chocolate mint water. ½ cup strawberries, ½ cup of pomegranate juice, and six leaves of chocolate mint.

Strawberry vanilla water. ½ cup strawberries, 1/8 tsp vanilla, two drops of stevia or monk fruit.

Tangerine cucumber water. 1 Tangerine sliced, 1/2 cucumber sliced.

Tarragon peach water. One sprig of tarragon, 1 cup peach sliced.

Vanilla orange water. One orange is sliced, one thin vanilla bean scraped or 1 tsp vanilla extract, 1 tsp of stevia or agave nectar or monk fruit.

Watermelon and basil: 1 cup fresh watermelon into small pieces with a few sprigs of fresh basil.

Watermelon basil water. One cup watermelon, six basil leaves.

Watermelon hibiscus water. One cup of watermelon 1 tsp hibiscus. You can find hibiscus in Whole Foods.

Watermelon jalapeno water. One cup watermelon, 1/2 cup fresh chopped jalapeno. Wear gloves to cut jalapeno.

Watermelon rosemary. One cup of watermelon, one sprig of rosemary.

Watermelon, kiwi, and lime. 1 cup watermelon, 1 kiwi diced or cut into circles, 1 lime sliced.

Ice cubes

If you don't want the taste of a full-blown natural flavored water, try adding some frozen blueberries or citrus zest to the water when you make your next batch of ice cubes. When frozen, you have little raw flavored cubes to pop in your water glass. They look fantastic and release and a nice flavor.

Fizzy water infusions

When you want that little bit of bubbly; just add seltzer water. It is best to make this by the glass; the bubbles won't last too long. You can use any of the above recipes to add to your seltzer water. You can also buy sparkling mineral water, it comes in many Citrus flavors, and you can add it to any of the recipes above.

Cilantro fizzy water. Three stems of cilantro, add seltzer water.

Sparkling Citrus. Using a squeeze of orange, lemon, or lime into sparkling mineral water.

Fennel fizzy water. 2 sprigs of fennel top in a glass of seltzer water.

Ginger Fizz. 1/4 inch peeled Ginger and seltzer water.

Hot water infusions

Hot infusions draw out vitamins, enzymes, and aromatic oils. A few good herbs for hot infusions include chamomile, basil, ginger, lavender nettle, peppermint, and skullcap.

To make a hot infusion drink, simply pour hot water over a certain amount of dried herb, covered, and steep.

There are many standard formulas for hot infusion; you can prepare individual servings and serve them hot or make a pitcher size and refrigerate.

Suggested equipment, tea pot, French press, tea ball infuser, reusable tea bags or cheesecloth.

It's easy to use a French press with any of the recipes listed below. You may need to adjust the number of ingredients based on your selected pot.

Lemon Ginger Infusion: Add 1-2 slices of fresh ginger and half a lemon to a cup of hot water. Steep for 5-10 minutes, and enjoy the tangy, refreshing flavor.

Mint Tea Infusion: Steep a handful of fresh mint leaves in hot water for 5-10 minutes. This infusion is perfect for digestion and relaxation.

Chamomile and Lavender Infusion: Mix 1 tablespoon each of dried chamomile and lavender flowers in a tea strainer and steep in hot water for 5-10 minutes. This infusion is known to promote sleep and relaxation.

Cinnamon and Apple Infusion: Add 1 cinnamon stick and a few slices of fresh apple to a cup of hot water. Steep for 5-10 minutes and enjoy a delicious, warming flavor.

Turmeric and Honey Infusion: Mix 1 teaspoon of turmeric powder and 1 teaspoon of honey in a cup of hot water. This infusion is known to boost the immune system and reduce inflammation.

Rose and Hibiscus Infusion: Mix 1 tablespoon each of dried rose petals and hibiscus flowers in a tea strainer and steep in hot water for 5-10 minutes. This infusion is rich in antioxidants and has a delicious floral flavor.

Lemon and Mint Infusion: Add 1-2 slices of fresh lemon and a handful of fresh mint leaves to a cup of hot water. Steep for 5-10 minutes, and enjoy a refreshing and citrusy taste.

Ginger and Turmeric Infusion: Mix 1 teaspoon each of ginger powder and turmeric powder in a cup of hot water. This infusion is known for its anti-inflammatory properties and can be enjoyed any time of day.

Peach and Mango Infusion: Add a few slices of fresh peach and mango to a cup of hot water. Steep for 5-10 minutes and enjoy a sweet and fruity flavor.

Blackberry and Sage Infusion: Mix 1 tablespoon of dried sage leaves and a handful of fresh blackberries in a tea strainer and steep in hot water for 5-10 minutes. This infusion is known to be high in antioxidants and has a unique, earthy flavor.

Chamomile Lavender Infusion: Add 1 tablespoon of dried chamomile flowers and 1 tablespoon of dried lavender flowers to a cup of hot water. Let it steep for 10 minutes before drinking.

Cinnamon Cardamom Infusion: Add 1 cinnamon stick and 3 cardamom pods to a cup of hot water. Let it steep for 5 minutes before drinking.

Mint Lime Infusion: Add 1 tablespoon of fresh mint leaves and 1 lime slice to a cup of hot water. Let it steep for 5 minutes before drinking.

Raspberry Rosehip Infusion: Add 1 tablespoon of dried raspberry leaves and 1 tablespoon of dried rosehips to a cup of hot water. Let it steep for 10 minutes before drinking.

Sage Lemon Infusion: Add 1 tablespoon of fresh sage leaves and 1 lemon slice to a cup of hot water. Let it steep for 5 minutes before drinking.

Peppermint Eucalyptus Infusion: Add 1 tablespoon of fresh peppermint leaves and 1 tablespoon of dried eucalyptus leaves to a cup of hot water. Let it steep for 10 minutes before drinking.

WATER CONSERVATION

Sadly, over one billion people lack safe drinking water due to pollution or no sources. We must take care of this precious resource so that future generations can enjoy it too. Of all the water on Earth, less than three percent is available for drinking, irrigation, and other uses.

Furthermore, only six countries contain more than half of the world's freshwater resources! As a result, more than a billion people do not have access to safe, clean water, and the number of thirsty people is increasing.

Further investigation of practical approaches and initiatives that can mitigate this critical situation and offer long-term solutions for communities requiring assistance.

1. Raising Awareness and Promoting Education: a. Educating communities: Implementing comprehensive education programs to raise awareness about water

pollution, sanitation practices, and sustainable water management. b. Advocacy campaigns: Engaging governments, non-profit organizations, and the media to promote awareness of the water crisis and foster global support for action.

2. Strengthening Water Infrastructure: a. Infrastructure development: Investing in the construction of water treatment facilities, pipelines, and distribution networks to provide safe drinking water to affected regions. b. Rainwater harvesting: Encouraging the adoption of rainwater collection systems in areas where water sources are scarce, thereby reducing reliance on polluted or limited sources.
3. Mitigating Pollution and Contamination: a. Industrial regulations: Implementing stringent regulations and monitoring mechanisms to control industrial pollution and enforce proper waste management practices. b. Agricultural practices: Promoting sustainable farming techniques, such as precision irrigation and organic farming, to minimize chemical runoff and water pollution.
4. Harnessing Innovative Technologies: a. Water purification systems: Deploying affordable and scalable water filtration technologies, such as reverse osmosis and UV disinfection, to remove contaminants and pathogens from polluted water sources. b. Mobile water treatment units: Utilizing portable treatment units

equipped with advanced purification technologies to provide immediate relief during emergencies and in remote areas lacking infrastructure.

5. Community Empowerment and Local Solutions: a. Empowering communities: Engaging local residents in the planning and implementation of water projects, ensuring their active involvement and ownership for long-term sustainability. b. Community-based water management: Promoting community-led initiatives, like water cooperatives or water user associations, to manage and protect water sources effectively.

By combining these strategies, we can work towards providing safe drinking water to over one billion people affected by pollution or limited water sources. Collaboration between governments, organizations, and individuals is crucial in implementing these solutions and fostering a future where clean and accessible water is a fundamental right for all.

Empowering Communities and Preserving a Precious Resource

Water is a fundamental resource for all life forms on Earth, and yet billions of people around the world still lack access to clean water. The scarcity of clean water poses a significant challenge, necessitating our collective responsibility to conserve water and ensure its sustainable management. By implementing various water conservation strategies and raising awareness about the importance of responsible water usage, we can contribute to alleviating the global water crisis and providing access to clean water for those in need. This article explores the significance of conserving water, highlights the challenges faced by communities without clean water, and provides practical ways individuals and societies can make a difference.

Understanding the Importance of Water Conservation

1. Ecological Balance: Water plays a vital role in maintaining ecological balance by sustaining ecosystems, supporting plant and animal life, and preserving biodiversity. By conserving water, we protect these delicate ecosystems and their inhabitants.
2. Health and Sanitation: Access to clean water is essential for human health and sanitation. Lack of clean water leads to the spread of waterborne diseases, resulting in illness and even death. By conserving water, we can reduce the burden of disease and improve public health.
3. Energy Conservation: Water and energy are closely interconnected. The energy required to extract, treat, and distribute water is significant. By conserving water, we indirectly conserve energy and reduce greenhouse gas emissions associated with water-related processes.

Challenges Faced by Communities Without Clean Water

1. Limited Access: Billions of people worldwide lack access to clean water, forcing them to rely on unsafe water sources such as rivers, ponds, or contaminated wells. This scarcity affects their daily lives, health, and economic opportunities.
2. Poverty and Inequality: Many communities lacking access to clean water are also affected by poverty and inequality. The burden of fetching water falls disproportionately on women and children, impacting their education, employment opportunities, and overall quality of life.
3. Water Stress and Climate Change: Water stress, caused by factors such as population growth, urbanization, and climate change, exacerbates the scarcity of water resources in various regions. Droughts, floods, and irregular rainfall patterns further challenge communities' access to clean water.

Practical Ways to Conserve Water

1. Raise Awareness: Education and awareness programs are crucial for promoting water conservation. By sharing information about the global water crisis, the importance of responsible water usage, and the impacts of individual actions, we can inspire behavioral change.

2. Reduce Household Consumption: Simple adjustments in daily routines can significantly reduce water usage. Install water-saving fixtures, repair leaks promptly, and adopt water-efficient practices such as taking shorter showers, turning off faucets while brushing teeth, and using dishwashers and washing machines efficiently.
3. Optimize Irrigation: In agricultural contexts, adopting water-efficient irrigation techniques such as drip irrigation, mulching, and crop rotation can reduce water waste. Farmers can also employ technologies like soil moisture sensors to optimize water usage based on crop needs.
4. Harvest and Reuse Water: Implement rainwater harvesting systems to capture and store rainwater for various purposes like irrigation, toilet flushing, and cleaning. Similarly, graywater recycling systems can treat and reuse water from sinks, showers, and laundry, minimizing overall water consumption.
5. Promote Water-Efficient Industries: Encourage industries to adopt water-saving technologies and practices, such as recycling and reusing water in manufacturing processes, as well as implementing efficient cooling and cleaning systems.
6. Support Community Initiatives: Support organizations working to provide access to clean water in underserved communities. Donate to initiatives building wells, water

treatment facilities, and sanitation infrastructure, and volunteer to assist in their implementation.

How Can You Help Conserve Our Precious Resource?

Conserving water is essential for both environmental sustainability and personal responsibility. Here are some specific actions individuals can take to conserve water:

1. Fix leaks: Regularly check for and promptly repair any leaks in faucets, toilets, and pipes. A dripping faucet can waste a significant amount of water over time.
2. Install water-efficient fixtures: Replace old, inefficient toilets, showerheads, and faucets with low-flow alternatives. These fixtures use less water while still maintaining adequate performance.
3. Take shorter showers: Aim to reduce your shower time by a few minutes. Consider using a shower timer or playing music to help you keep track and make it a habit.
4. Turn off faucets: When brushing your teeth, shaving, or washing dishes, turn off the faucet when not actively using the water. This simple step can save several gallons of water per minute.
5. Use a bucket for rinsing: When washing fruits, vegetables, or dishes, place a basin or bucket in the sink to collect the initial cold water. You can reuse this water for plants or other purposes.

6. Opt for full loads: Utilize dishwashers and washing machines only when you have a full load of dishes or laundry. This maximizes water efficiency and reduces the number of cycles needed.
7. Capture rainwater: Install rain barrels or tanks to collect rainwater from gutters and downspouts. This water can be used for watering plants, cleaning outdoor areas, or even flushing toilets.
8. Mulch and water efficiently: Apply a layer of mulch around plants and trees to retain moisture and reduce evaporation. Water plants during the cooler hours of the day to minimize water loss through evaporation.
9. Reuse water: Reuse water from activities like rinsing fruits and vegetables, or leftover drinking water, to water indoor or outdoor plants.
10. Use a broom, not a hose: Instead of using a hose to clean outdoor areas like patios or driveways, sweep them with a broom. This not only saves water but also avoids unnecessary runoff.
11. Adjust sprinklers and irrigation: Regularly check your sprinkler system for leaks, and make sure it is properly adjusted to avoid watering sidewalks or driveways. Consider installing a rain sensor to prevent unnecessary watering during rainy periods.
12. Consider xeriscaping: If possible, choose drought-tolerant plants for your garden that require less water. Implement xeriscaping techniques such as grouping

plants with similar water needs together and using efficient irrigation methods.

13. Educate yourself and others: Stay informed about water conservation practices and spread awareness among family, friends, and community members. Encourage them to adopt water-saving habits as well.

Remember, every drop counts, and by implementing these specific water conservation practices, you can make a significant impact in preserving this precious resource.

My Final Thoughts

As we wrap up the wonders of "The Miracle Molecule," it's unmistakable how central water is to, well, everything. The story of water is the story of life. It's there in every cell, every breath, and every heartbeat, keeping our bodies on the go and literally shaping the world around us. It's been eye-opening to see just how interconnected we are with the natural cycle of water, from the rain that feeds our crops to the rivers that power our cities.

Then there's this whole fascinating idea of water memory, suggesting that water isn't just a passive carrier of life but an active participant in our health and happiness. It's a bit out there, sure, but it's thrilling to think about the implications, about how staying hydrated could be as much about nourishing our spirit as our cells.

It's not just about drinking enough water (though, seriously, don't skimp on that). It's about stepping up and taking care of this incredible resource that takes care of us. Whether it's cutting down on waste, protecting natural waterways, or just being a bit more mindful about how we use water, it's on us to make a difference.

So, as we close this chapter (pun intended), I'm hope you have a renewed awe for the humble molecule that sustains us all. Water isn't just something we consume; it's something we're a part of. It's a reminder to not only cherish and protect the water around us but also to appreciate the flow of life it enables within us.

Here's to water—may we never take it for granted, but instead honor it as the priceless treasure it is. Let's pledge to be stewards of our water, for our sake and for the planet's. Remember, every little bit helps, so let's make every drop count.

REFERENCES

Murray RK, Granner DK, Mayes PA, Rodwell VW. (2006). Harper's Illustrated Biochemistry. New York: Lange Medical Books/McGraw-Hill.

Ginès P, Schrier RW. (2003). Renal Failure in Cirrhosis. The New England Journal of Medicine, 349: 830-839.

Thompson C, Wistrom J, Gosink J. (2008). Dehydration Impairs Performance and Impacts Biochemical Markers. International Journal of Sports Medicine, 29(02):111-118.

MKohlmeier@Forefrontderm.com. "The Role Water Plays in Skin Health." Forefront Dermatology, 21 Mar. 2018, forefrontdermatology.com/role-water-plays-skin-health.

Groth, Leah, and Mohiba Tareen MD. "Can You Hydrate Your Way to Healthy Skin?" EverydayHealth.com, 25 May 2023, www.everydayhealth.com/healthy-skin/can-you-hydrate-your-way-to-healthy-skin.

How Drinking Water Helps Your Skin and Hair. Multipure, www.multipure.com/purely-social/science/how-drinking-water-helps-skin. Accessed 27 May 2023.

Popkin, B. M., D'Anci, K. E., & Rosenberg, I. H. (2010). Water, Hydration, and Health. *Nutrition Reviews*, 68(8), 439–458. This comprehensive review discusses the role of water in human physiology, including its effects on function and health.

Jéquier, E., & Constant, F. (2010). Water as an essential nutrient: the physiological basis of hydration. *European Journal of Clinical Nutrition*, 64, 115–123. This article explains water's critical roles in the human body, emphasizing its necessity for physical and mental performance.

Armstrong, L. E. (2007). Assessing hydration status: the elusive gold standard. *Journal of the American College of Nutrition*, 26(sup5), 575S-584S. This paper evaluates methods for assessing hydration and discusses the physiological impact of fluid balance.

Kleiner, S. M. (1999). Water: an essential but overlooked nutrient. *Journal for the American Dietetic Association*, 99(2), 200-206. This article underscores water's critical role in nutrition and health maintenance.

Sawka, M. N., Cheuvront, S. N., & Carter, R. (2005). Human water needs. *Nutrition Reviews*, 63(s1), S30-S39. This research provides an overview of human water requirements and hydration's effects on health.

Perrier, E. T., Buendia-Jimenez, I., Vecchio, M., Armstrong, L. E., Tack, I., & Klein, A. (2015). Twenty-four-hour urine osmolality as a physiological index of adequate water intake. *Disease Markers*, 2015. This study suggests urinary markers for determining adequate hydration levels.

Stookey, J. D., Constant, F., Popkin, B. M., & Gardner, C. D. (2008). Drinking water is associated with weight loss in overweight dieting women independent of diet and activity. *Obesity*, 16(11), 2481-2488. This observational study links higher water consumption with weight loss efforts.

Pross, N. (2017). Effects of Dehydration and Rehydration on Cognitive Performance and Mood. *Nutrition Reviews*, 72(suppl 2), 144-154. This paper reviews the cognitive and mood changes associated with hydration status changes.

Boschmann, M., Steiniger, J., Hille, U., Tank, J., Adams, F., Sharma, A. M., Klaus, S., Luft, F. C., & Jordan, J. (2003). Water-induced thermogenesis. *The Journal of Clinical Endocrinology & Metabolism*, 88(12), 6015-6019. This study explores how drinking water can increase energy expenditure.

Manz, F., & Wentz, A. (2005). The importance of good hydration for the prevention of chronic diseases. *Nutrition Reviews*, 63(suppl 1), S2-S5. This comprehensive review links adequate hydration with chronic disease prevention, including urinary tract infections and hypertension.

Dennis, E. A., Dengo, A. L., Comber, D. L., Flack, K. D., Savla, J., Davy, K. P., & Davy, B. M. (2010). Water consumption increases weight loss during a hypocaloric diet intervention in middle-aged and older adults. *Obesity*, 18(2), 300-307. This study demonstrates that increased water consumption is associated with enhanced weight loss in individuals undergoing a calorie-restricted diet.

Bar-David, Y., Urkin, J., & Kozminsky, E. (2005). The effect of voluntary dehydration on cognitive functions of elementary school children. *Acta Paediatrica*, 94(11), 1667-1673. This research investigates how dehydration negatively impacts cognitive functions in children.

Spigt, M. G., Knottnerus, J. A., Westerterp, K. R., Olde Rikkert, M. G., & Schayck, C. P. (2006). Increasing the daily water intake for the prophylactic treatment of headache: a pilot trial. *European Journal of Neurology*, 13(9), 954-958. This pilot study explores how increasing daily water intake can reduce the frequency and intensity of headaches.

Edmonds, C. J., Jeffes, B. (2009). Does having a drink help you think? 6–7-year-old children show improvements in cognitive performance from baseline to test after having a drink of water. *Appetite*, 53(3), 469-472. This study highlights the immediate cognitive benefits of hydration in young children.

Chang, T., Ravi, N., Plegue, M. A., Sonneville, K. R., & Davis, M. M. (2016). Inadequate Hydration, BMI, and Obesity Among US Adults: NHANES 2009-2012. *Annals of Family Medicine*, 14(4), 320-324. This research correlates inadequate hydration with higher BMI and obesity rates in U.S. adults.

Made in the USA
Monee, IL
03 November 2026

67384074R00128